EPIGMENIO CASTILLO GALLEGOSS
ELIAZAR OCAÑA ZAVALETA
BRAULIO VALLES DE LA MORA

Arachis pintoi, an alternative in cattle feeding

EPIGMENIO CASTILLO GALLEGOSS
ELIAZAR OCAÑA ZAVALETA
BRAULIO VALLES DE LA MORA

Arachis pintoi, an alternative in cattle feeding

Arachis pintoi as a sustainable and sustainable system for cattle feeding in the humid tropics of Mexico.

ScienciaScripts

Imprint

Any brand names and product names mentioned in this book are subject to trademark, brand or patent protection and are trademarks or registered trademarks of their respective holders. The use of brand names, product names, common names, trade names, product descriptions etc. even without a particular marking in this work is in no way to be construed to mean that such names may be regarded as unrestricted in respect of trademark and brand protection legislation and could thus be used by anyone.

Cover image: www.ingimage.com

This book is a translation from the original published under ISBN 978-620-2-11003-7.

Publisher:
Sciencia Scripts
is a trademark of
Dodo Books Indian Ocean Ltd. and OmniScriptum S.R.L publishing group

120 High Road, East Finchley, London, N2 9ED, United Kingdom
Str. Armeneasca 28/1, office 1, Chisinau MD-2012, Republic of Moldova, Europe
Printed at: see last page
ISBN: 978-620-5-60360-4

Copyright © EPIGMENIO CASTILLO GALLEGOSS, ELIAZAR OCAÑA ZAVALETA, BRAULIO VALLES DE LA MORA
Copyright © 2023 Dodo Books Indian Ocean Ltd. and OmniScriptum S.R.L publishing group

INDEX

CHAPTER I

Population dynamics of Arachis pintoi CIAT17434, associated with native grasses under grazing in the humid tropics of Mexico.

Lidia Ascencio Rojas, Epigmenio Castillo Gallegos, Braulio Valles de la Mora"†"

INTRODUCTION

Production in the tropics has increased in recent decades as a result of the green revolution, which consisted of the intensification of production through the use of large quantities of inputs such as fertilizers, improved varieties and crop protection. The tropical pasture revolution emerged in the 1960s and resulted in a significant increase in livestock food production potential (Mennetje, 1995).The intensification of livestock systems is normally accompanied by the use of chemical nitrogen fertilizers, but these can be substituted by nitrogen biologically fixed by leguminous plants associated with existing grasses in the pasture, which can lead to an increase in biomass production (CATIE, 1990) and to the survival of species under grazing. To understand the mechanisms of survival of species under grazing. It is necessary to implement studies on population dynamics (Mennetje 1989).Traditionally, animal production systems in the Mexican tropics are based on the use of native forage species of low productivity and marked seasonality, both in production and quality (Ramos, 1983). Grazing is continuous and the survival of the botanical components is guaranteed due to this conservative management; however, when the intention is to intensify animal production, introduced forage species are used, both as grasses and legumes; but in the case of the latter, their permanence in the field is short, mainly due to the poor The ability to resist grazing and trampling, in addition to the low tolerance to competition with more aggressive species (Humphereys, 1989). Arachis pintoi has been noted for its persistence under grazing, but its mechanisms of survival under grazing are not fully understood to date, so this study aims to provide a minimum of basic knowledge of these mechanisms, in order to improve the management of these species under Mexican humid tropical conditions (Grof, 1985).

LITERATURE REVIEW

Importance of forages in Mexican livestock.
Role of forages in Mexican livestock.

Cattle raising in the tropics is sustained by the forage resources of these areas, because the characteristics of the climate (abundant rainfall and high temperatures mainly), soil and topography are more favorable for grazing than for the cultivation of agricultural products, so that the tropics are considered as eminently cattle-raising areas, where an important meat production industry has developed in which forage, consumed in direct grazing, constitutes the basis of the most economical feeding of ruminants (Valles, 1984).The sustainability of associated grass-legume forage species depends on the persistence of both components, which in turn depends on the environment and management. The latter mainly encompasses fertilization and defoliation by cutting or grazing. Grazing management has two main components, stocking rate and grazing method (mannentje, 1995).

Role of forages in Mexican livestock.

The latter mainly encompasses fertilization and defoliation by cutting or grazing (McWilliam, 1978), since soil moisture deficiency affects The use of this product is a significant growth promoter and promotes the rapid dehydration of forage species.On the other hand, adequate seed production is also important for the development and persistence of forage species Cruz et al. (1999), mention that high seed production can ensure the survival of forage species to adverse factors, such as drought, severe winters and overgrazing.The importance of associating productive legumes to native pastures in the tropics is due to their potential to improve the quality of the animal's diet and add organic matter and nitrogen to the soil, maintaining or increasing its fertility (Monsalve, 2000), which would allow for the sustainability of dual-purpose livestock farming. Research carried out since 1987 at CEIEGT (Centro de Enseñanza e Investigación en Ganadería Tropical) indicated that the herbaceous legume Arachis pintoi CIAT 17434, known as forage peanut, is an option for pasture improvement, since it is persistent and aggressive when associated with grasses that are also aggressive, both native and improved (Hernández et al., 1990; Arzola et al., 1997).

Native grasses: The basis of livestock feed for grazing.

Because of the area they cover, grasses are the most important food resource in the humid tropics of Mexico, but their forage quality and production are poor to fair, which can be accentuated by the inefficient management they receive. This is one of the reasons why the legume Arachis pintoi was introduced to native grass pastures in an attempt to improve forage quality and production, as well as milk production and soil fertility (Castillo, 2000). Experimental work has been carried out in this same region that has highlighted the important role of introduced legumes when associated with native grasses. The main benefit indicates an improvement in diet quality and milk production (Chantal, 1998).

Description of Arachis pintoi legumes

Arachis pintoi is a legume native to Brazil (Valls and Simpson, 1993) that has become popular among avant-garde farmers in the humid tropics of Latin America, because it adapts to acid soils of low fertility in this region and competes efficiently for stable associations with grasses (Ibrahim, 1994); in addition, it has shown good performance in agronomic evaluations (Vall and Pizarro, 1994).Arachis pintoi is a herbaceous perennial plant with creeping and stoloniferous growth, taproot, taproot and alternate compound leaves with four leaflets, slightly flattened stem with short interknots and yellow flower is a geocarpic plant with single-seeded pods formed at the end of the gynophore (Cook et al., 1980).The legume has a wide range of adaptation, but grows well in tropical conditions between 0 and 1800 meters above sea level. And with a total annual rainfall of 2000 to 3500 mm well distributed throughout the year. It grows in a wide range of soils with texture varying from clay to sandy. It adapts well to acid soils with high aluminum saturation (70%) or more but grows on soils with more than 3% organic matter (Azakawa and Ramirez, 1989). This legume does not tolerate drought, this should not be more than 3 to 4 months, it can maintain green stolons retaining a good proportion of foliage; at the beginning of the rains, the seed stored in the soil germinates with great vigor (CIAT, 1997).Arachis pintoi has a great capacity to associate with forage grasses, due to its propagation by stolons, high persistence under grazing, good quality and consumption by animals. Therefore, this legume has a high potential to improve animal production and the physical and chemical conditions of the soil (Rincón, Arguelles, 1991).Although this species flowers prolifically, little is known about the efficiency of seed formation (Ferguson, 1995). The species can regenerate from seed, or rhizomes and stolons, which contributes to its ability to persist and resist inadequate management (Fisher and Cruz, 1995). Thus, unlike what happens with creeping plants, the damage or fracture to the plant by animal hooves is insignificant (Fisher and Cruz, 1995). Photo. 1, 2, and 3.

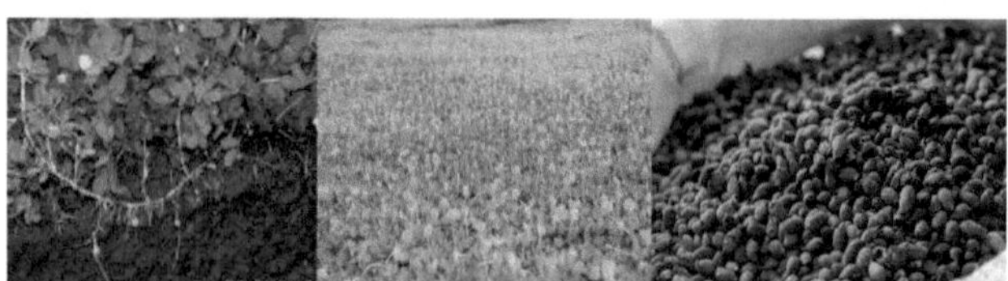

Photo. 1. A. pintoi stolons Photo 2. Flower of A. pintoi Photo. 3. A. pintoi seeds.

What is population density?

Population dynamics or plant demography is related to the number of plants in the meadow or how these numbers combine over time (Harper, 1977).The most important plant survival factors are those related to the appearance and death of individuals at any time. The population density depends on the change in the number of incoming and outgoing individuals.Such changes are always occurring, even in botanically stable forage species, for example, some stolons of pangola grass (Digitaria decumbens) would be dying when new stolons are forming. It is also possible to obtain annually stable grasslands in the sense that the botanical composition is similar from one year to another, despite the fact that the biological cycle of the plants, their growth and the formation of new stolons is repeated year after year.of seeds. Poor persistence implies poor regeneration (Harper, 1978).When planting a species in a prepared field, there is a reasonable chance of achieving a desired population density by manipulating the planting density and timing of planting. The probability of success decreases with broadcast seeding, but in general, newly introduced species constitute a population where all seedlings become established at virtually the same time. However, all of these plants may die (Harper, 1978).

Persistence mechanism

The persistence mechanisms of plants in the field depend to a great extent on several factors. Some of the most important are described below.

Flowering

The process of seed formation is highly dependent on soil temperature and moisture availability, in addition to the effect of photoperiod. On the other hand, animal stocking exerts the greatest effect on flowering and seed production compared to other management factors. Grazing not only defoliates plants but also eliminates growing points and in doing so, also eliminates inflorescence formation points (Mannentje, 1996).

Stolon density

Stoloniferous and rhizomatous species do not depend exclusively on flowering and seed production for their regeneration, as is the case of some leguminous plants such as Trifolium repends, Desmodium ovalifolium Arachis glabrata, Desmodium hetereophyllum and Arachis pintoi (Jones and Carter, 1989). The aforementioned species reproduce on stolons, and the new plants are develop from the stolon nodes. The density and length of the stolons are considered as an agronomic characteristic that explains, in part, the longevity of the species in the field, so their study is considered of primary importance. Photos 4, 5, 6, 7 and 8.

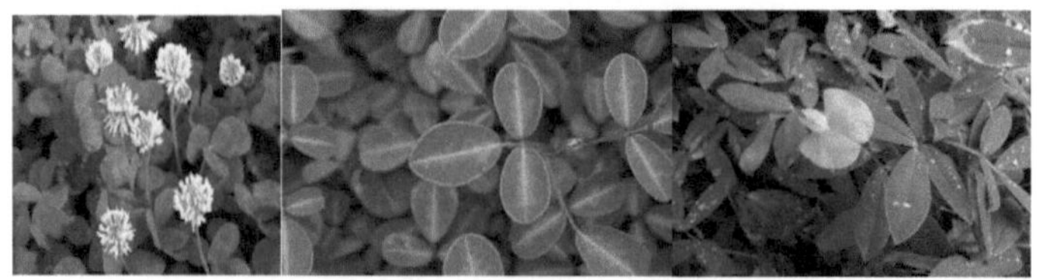

Photo. 4. Trifolium repends Photo. 5. Desmodium ovalifolium Photo.6. Arachis glabrata

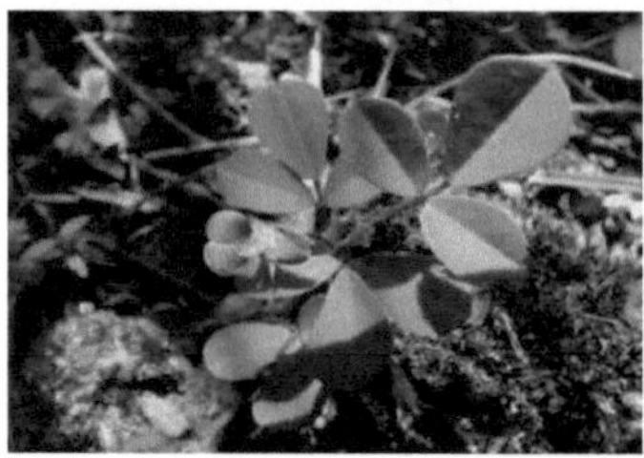

Photo .7. Desmodium hetereophyllum

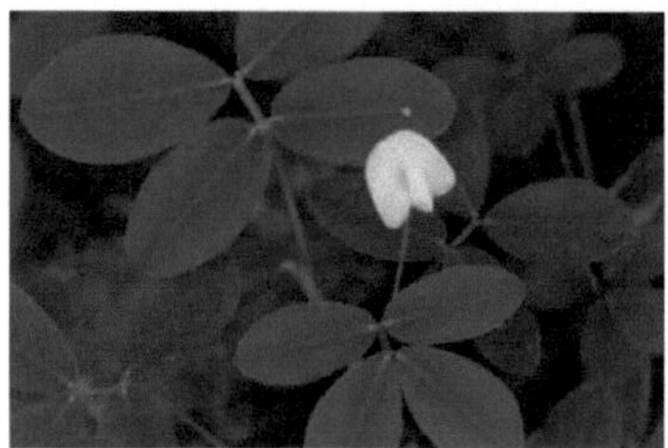

Photo .8. Arachis pintoi

In addition, the high stolon development of Arachis pintoi up to 555 stolons/ m^2 at three months of age under humid tropical conditions favors soil conservation programs (CIAT, 1990).

Germination

Viable and softened seeds that are not deeply buried germinate when temperature and humidity conditions are favorable. The main cause of seed death is, therefore, soil water deficit, in regions with variable rainfall, it is advantageous for the persistence of the legume, the occurrence of waves of germination during the rains, since a seed stock with several The age of the plants has a better chance of becoming established and developing into adult plants (Mannetje et al., 1983).

Weather

Forage production in tropical zones is characterized by its marked seasonality, as a result of climatic variations during the year. Thus, in the tropical region of the Gulf of Mexico, the climatic succession of drought (March-June), summer (July-October) and winter (November-February) (Hernández et al. 1990) determines to a great extent forage production and its quality, and also affects to a great extent forage production and its quality, as well as the survival mechanisms of plants, such as seed formation, stolon elongation and growing points.For a population to survive, dying plants must be replaced by new plants. The appearance of new plants can occur by sexual or asexual processes. For a forage species to persist through asexual reproduction, it must produce seed as long as it has been grazed, since the amount of dormant seed remaining from the original seeding is generally very low (Mannetje et al., 1995).

Some species, such as Stylosanthes sp photo 9, reproduce only sexually while Pangola grass, photo 10, a sterile grass, reproduces only asexually. Other species such as white clover, Trifolium repens photo. 11, can persist by both mechanisms. In these species the relative importance of each mechanism may vary with management or climatic conditions. For example: White clover tends to persist in the Australian subtropics by seedling regeneration on drier sites or in years with more drought, or by stolons on wet sites or in wet years (Jones, 1982).

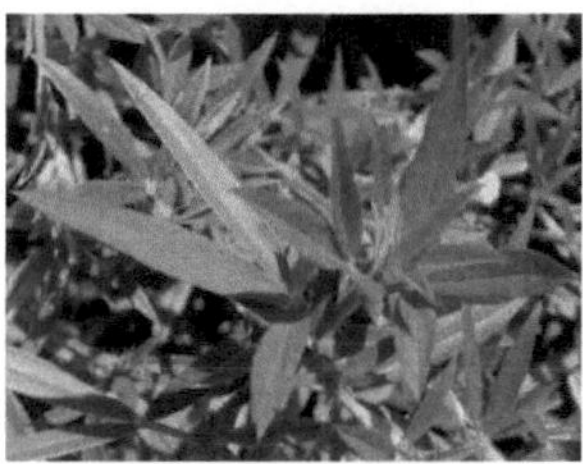

Photo. 9 Stylosanthes sp

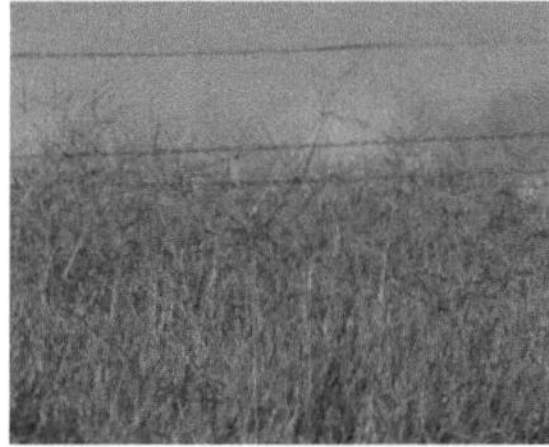

Photo 10. Pangola Digitaria d

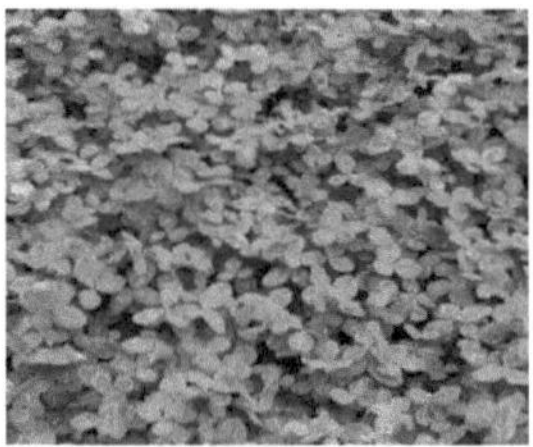

Photo. 11Trifolium repens

Since the tracking of new plants by sexual reproduction depends on seed production, it is important to consider the various ways in which seeds can be lost from their formation in the plant growing in the pasture to the successful establishment of a seedling. It is easy to overlook seed loss through predation, an activity that can become very intense.For example (Gardener, 1982), in California in a meadow he observed that 75% of fescue was consumed by rodents. This author suggested that in general animals are the main cause of seed loss in temperate perennial grasslands.

Plant characteristics related to persistence:

Hodgkinson and Williams (1983) have listed several characteristics that favor plant survival under grazing conditions. Some of these are:

1. Position of basal meristems of prostrate leaves and stems.

2. Firm anchorage of the roots.

3. Shoot formation from the roots.

4. Rapid onset of meristems.

5. Appearance of latency during drought

6. Appearance of floral structures close to the ground.

7. Fast playback.

8. Seed burial mechanisms.

9. Retention of seed variability excreted in feces. 10 Formation of hard seeds.
11. Morphological and biochemical deterrents.

The most resistant plants present some, but not all of these attributes; for example, seed burial mechanisms are important for the persistence of some species, but are not present in Stylosanthes species which, even so, can be very persistent (Hodgkinson and Williams, 1983). Pueraria phaseloydes (Kudzú) photo 12, presents the problem of low survival under intensive grazing, because its growing points are located within reach of cattle, therefore its persistence in the pasture is threatened under such management; thus defoliation has very negative effects on the survival of plants, if their regenerative points are destroyed, or a reduction in the root system increases the susceptibility of plants to drought, diseases or insect damage (Humphreys, 1991).

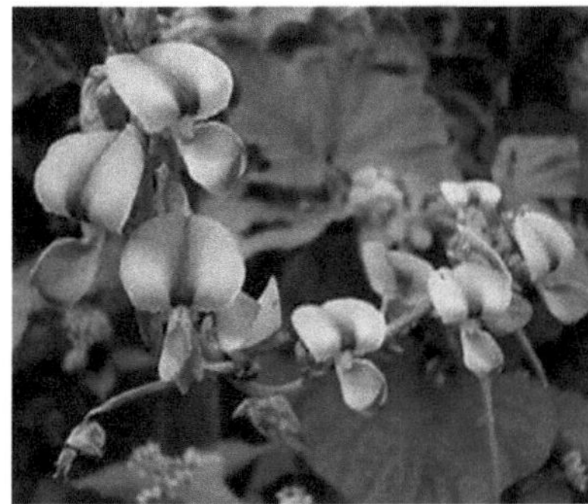

Photo 12.Pueraria phaseloydes (Kudzú).

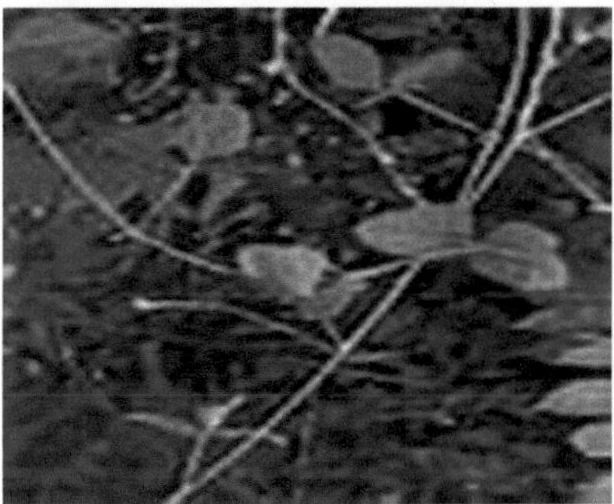

Photo 13 Microptilium atropurpureum.

Under extreme weather conditions (severe winter or drought), reserve photosynthates may be important to ensure the permanence of the species in the field (Harris, 1978). NMicroptilium atropurpureum, photo 13, resprouts from the crown and stolons, new plants emerge from seeds in the soil, precipitation and grazing pressure affect the longevity and reproductive form of this species (Jones and Buch, 1988). When precipitation is high, roots form from nodes, which favors the emergence of new plants. This does not occur in dry seasons when reserve seeds in the soil are the only form of regeneration (Jones and Mannentje, 1986).High pressure reduces the persistence and seed production of forage plants, decreasing their reserve in the soil and contributing to the disappearance of species. The stoloniferous and prostrate species of Desmodium heterophyllium, photo 14, tolerate high animal loads due to the effect of their growing points at soil level, being potentially persistent to the associations (Mannentje, 1989). Such is the case, for example, of the grasses of the genera photo. 15 Setaria and photo. 16 Paspalum, where the presence of carbohydrates in the plant was associated with tolerance to low temperatures.

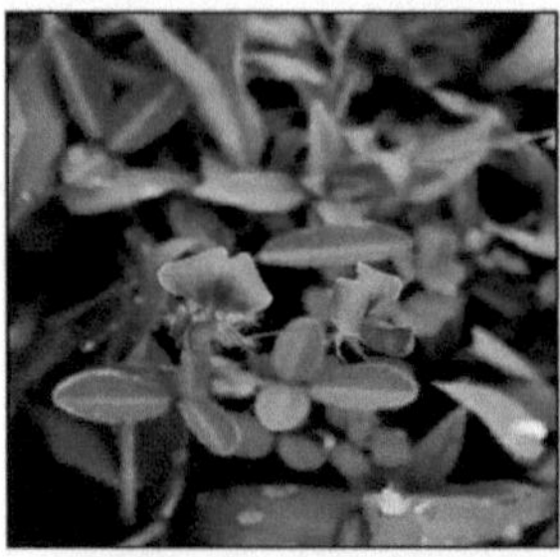

Photo 14 Desmodium heterophyllium.

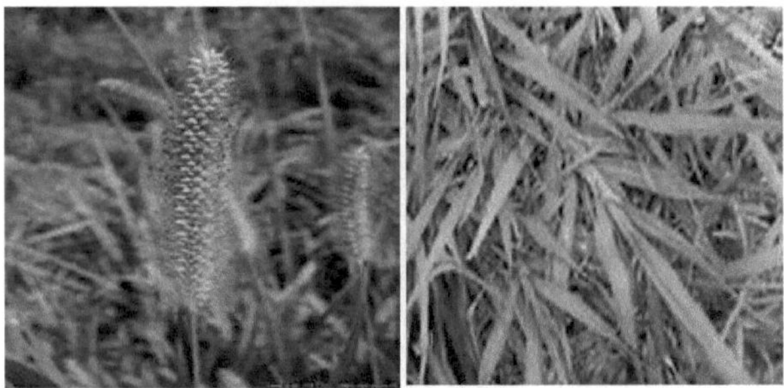

Photo 15.Setaria. sp.
Photo. 16 Paspalum.ssp.

Plant survival

There is little information on long-term studies that have evaluated the survivability of Arachis pintoi, even though this species has been evaluated in the last few years. is a requirement for designing grazing management programs that allow the persistence of desirable species (Jones and Carter, 1989).This is due to the limited application of biological principles by forage specialists; in addition, measurements are tedious and require long periods of time to be reliable (Mannetje, 1995). However, demographic studies of forage species are necessary because they help to predict the effects of management and its relationship with climate on the persistence of the species under study. Likewise, they allow to know the characteristics of the plant that help to its persistence, allow the creation of growth models of forage species subject to grazing, with which phytogeneticists design selection and genetic

10

improvement programs. In addition, with some basic knowledge, the extensionist can incorporate demographic information into his consultancies (Jones and Carter, 1989).

Factors influencing the persistence of grasslands.

Factors such as site and all management factors can influence the persistence of grasslands. Environmental factors include soil type, slope, drainage, rainfall and distribution, pests and diseases, and in some cases burning. Many of these factors cannot be controlled under normal management conditions. If a higher economic return is expected from forage crops, then environmental conditions can be modified through operations such as irrigation and pest control (Mackeon and Mott, 1984).The management factors of a pasture are mainly the duration and intensity of grazing, soil fertility that can be modified by fertilizer application and burning.Some practical reasons for studying persistence mechanisms are first to understand how environmental factors affect persistence processes, and how plants respond to management factors (grazing type, stocking rate, mowing) McKeon and Mott, 1984).

Role of the seed reserve in the soil

The presence of seeds in the soil guarantees the persistence of the species in the field (Cruz et al., 1999). Thus, seed production is a desirable characteristic in the process of selection of forage materials, both for commercial production and to ensure the natural seeding of pastures. In all cases, it is sought that the production be abundant, with good quality seed and high viability. Flowering and subsequent seed formation depend to a great extent on favorable climatic conditions. Numerous observations indicate that severe droughts negatively affect seed production, since moisture stress reduces the flowering rate of forage species (Rossiter, 1978); it has also been observed that photoperiod affects the flowering process and seed formation (Humphreys, 1981).In the case of Arachis pintoi, they indicated that this species requires between 12 to 18 months to reach maximum seed production, and mentioned that the range varies between 900 and 6000 kg, depending on environmental conditions and age of the crop (Argel and Pizarro, 1992), and that better soil fertility, with high calcium content, results in better harvests (Enriquez, 2001).

Contributions to the soil by leguminous plants

Leguminous plants such as Arachis pintoi can also increase soil fertility by incorporating nitrogen into the soil-plant-animal system through biological fixation. Studies carried out by Valles (2001) at CEIEGT indicated that 80% of the nitrogen contained in three accessions of Arachis pintoi (CIAT 17434, 18744 and 18748) came from biological fixation. At the same site, Castillo (2000) observed that, after 2 years of experimentation, the nitrogen content in the soil (0-20 cm) was 17 kg/ha in a pasture of native grasses, while in the association between native grasses and Arachis pintoi, the content was 32 kg/ha.

In addition, leguminous plants also contribute to soil fertility improvement through the supply of nutrients via decomposition of plant residues such as leaves, stems, roots and nodules (Cadisch et al., 1994).

Legume quality

It has been widely demonstrated that the nutritional quality of legumes is superior to that of grasses (Giller and Gilson, 1991: and in the case of Arachis pintoi, at CEIEGT Sosa (2001) determined in situ digestibility values higher than 65% and crude protein contents in the range of 10-16% in forage ingested by dual-purpose cows fistulated to the esophagus. The botanical composition of this forage comprised 22% Arachis pintoi and 78% grasses.

Animal production

In the humid tropics of Costa Rica, Arachis pintoi associated with Brachiaria grasses, showed the capacity to improve the production of 6 to 8 kg/cow/day (Van Heurch, 1990), as well as the weight gain of steers, registering a production of 987 kg/ha/year (Ibrahim, 1994). This is a record for crops without irrigation and fertilization.In the Mexican tropics, under extensive grazing conditions, meat yields of 380 to 672 kg/ha/year have been achieved, depending on the species associations (Enriquez and Castillo, 1996). With the use of grasses and legumes and good pasture management, it has been possible to achieve animal yields of more than 600 g/day with tropical pastures (Milera, 1991). In zebu cattle, live weight gains of 92, 143, 148 kg/ha/year have been achieved with stocking rates of 5.0, 3.6 and 2.8 AU/ha (Lazcano and Avila, 1991).Milk production per cow in legume associations can be higher by almost 0.5 kg/day. In a study conducted by CIAT (1997) where cows of the Criollo Dairy and Jersey breeds were used, milk yields of 8.8, 7.7, 7.6 kg/cow/day were observed for the treatments of Arachis estrella de Santo Domingo (Cynodon nlemfuensis), Desmodium-estrella and estrella sola, respectively. Previously, Lascano and Avila (1991) reported yields of 9.5, 10.8 and 9.4 kg/ha/day for the same pastures, respectively.

Forage production

Grazing, in the north-central region of the state of Veracruz, is in the range of 28 kg DM/day, which is similar to the production of native grasses in the area (Gómez-Cortés et al., 1994). In Costa Rica, Hernandez et al., (1995) reported forage ranges at the beginning of grazing from 3.5 to tons DM/ha, depending on whether the applied stocking rate was high or low. In the same country. Ibrahim and Manneje (1988) reported values of 4 and 5 tons DM/ha for drought and rainy seasons, respectively, when changing the cutting frequency from 4 to 12 weeks.On the other hand, it is possible to find differences in forage production according to the accession in question; Villa Ruel and Zúñiga (1996) evaluated the accessions of Arachis pintoi

CIAT 17434, 18744 and 18748. They found that biomass production increased with age at cutting, being the annual increase of 6, 2 and 4.0 ton/MS/ha, respectively, when changing the cutting frequency from 4 to 12 weeks.

Native grasses

Native grasses are the main forage resource in the Mexican tropics, where they occupy up to 75% of the grazing land. Native grasses, traditionally with continuous grazing, have low annual productions, in the order of a ton of DM/ha, and their quality is regular to poor with a crude protein (CP) percentage of 4% to 7%, with a digestibility of 45 to 55%; therefore, their carrying capacity is between 1-1.5 animal units (AU/ha) (Minson, 1990). Intensive rotational management allows for an increase in the content of PC protein to the range of 7 to 14%, but digestibility as well as dry matter production remains low.The low forage yield is due to the fact that soil nutrients, mainly nitrogen, limit the growth of grasses during the year, particularly in the tropics, where ranchers are not accustomed to fertilize their pastures (Bosman et al., 1990). These pastures are mostly composed of Paspalum sp, Axonopus sp, and Cynodon sp, and to a lesser extent of Desmodium scorpiurus and Centrosema sp (Gómez-Cortés et al., 1994).

Justification of the study

Although Ibrahim (1994), observed that Arachis pintoi is a persistent and competitive species due to its short internodes and prostrate growth, which allow heavy grazing, to be able to regenerate from the soil seed reservoir, as well as rooting and stolon branching, his results came from a site with very fertile (> 10% organic matter) and deep soils (< 3 m) with abundant rainfall (< 3000 mm/year), high animal stocking, and slow rotation and beef cattle.10% organic matter) and deep (< 3 m) soils with abundant rainfall (< 3000 mm/year), high stocking rates, and with slow rotation and beef cattle.However, the conditions at CEIEGT are different, since intensive rotation with dual-purpose cows is managed there, on soil that is not very fertile (2% organic matter) and shallow (20 cm), with a tendency to waterlogging and rainfall of < 2000 mm/year.) The association of legumes to native pastures in the tropics promotes an improvement in the animals' diet, adding organic matter and nitrogen to the soil, maintaining or increasing its fertility, which allows dual-purpose livestock farming to become sustainable. These differences are sufficient reason to justify the study of Arachis pintoi plant demography under the prevailing conditions of CEIEGT.

Hypothesis

The high persistence of Arachis pintoi associated with native grasses (Paspalum sp), grazing, is given by survival mechanisms such as stolon density and rooting points, in addition to its abundant regeneration from the soil seed reservoir.

Objectives

1. To determine the degree of survival of Arachis pintoi plants in the association of this legume with native grasses.

2. To identify the survival mechanisms of Arachis pintoi under tropical, warm and humid climate conditions in the north-central region of the state of Veracruz.

3. To determine the survival mechanisms of Arachis pintoi associated with native grasses and under intensive rotational grazing with dual-purpose cows.

MATERIAL AND METHODS

Location of the study

The experimental phase was carried out at the Centro de Enseñanza, Investigación y Extensión en Ganadería Tropical CEIEGT) belonging to the Facultad de Medicina Veterinaria y Zootecnia of the Universidad Nacional Autónoma de México, located at Km.5.5 of the federal highway Martínez de la Torre-Tlapacoyan whose geographical location is 97° 06, west longitude, 20° 01· north latitude and 103 masl altitude. Koepen's climate classification, modified by García (1988) for Mexico, classifies the climate as Warm humid Af (m) W" (e), without a dry season. The mean annual temperature is 25.5 +0.5 +0.5⁰ C, the thermal oscillation is extreme from 7 to 14° C, and the mean annual precipitation is 1991 mm + 392 mm. The high coefficient of variation for monthly precipitation (50%) indicates low rainfall reliability. There are three climatic epochs: high precipitation and high temperatures (rainfall, July to October), low precipitation and low temperatures (north, November to February), and low precipitation and high temperatures (drought, March to June) (Toledo, 1989) Figure 1 presents the climatic conditions prevailing during the experimental period.

Type of soil

The soils originated from weathered sandstone from ancient alluvial sedimentation. Throughout the area there is a hard horizon of low permeability known locally as tepetate that occurs at depths between 5 and 25 cm. These soils are classified as Ultisols, Acidic (pH5.o 5.5), clayey, with low aluminum saturation, but increasing with depth (10.5%, 27.5%, and 31.3% for depths of 0-10 cm, 10-20 cm, 20-30 cm and 30 to 40 cm. Phosphorus, calcium sulfur and potassium levels are considered low (< 3ppm, < 30 ppm, 3 meq/100g. 0.2 Meq/100, respectively) and the organic matter content at a depth of 0-10 cm is of medium range, around 3% (Toledo, 1989).

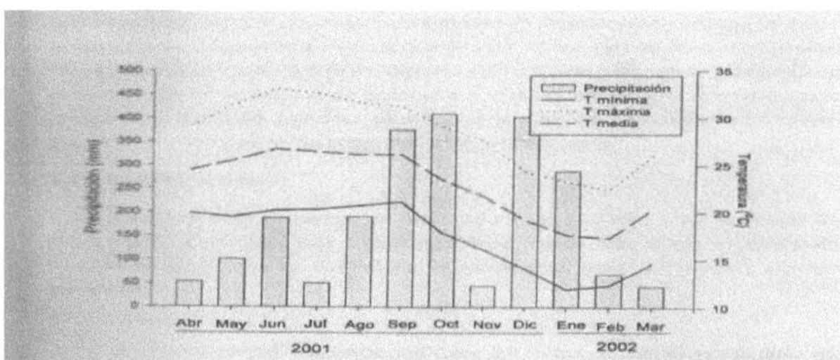

Figure 1. Temperature y precipitation at a climate warm humid Tlapacoyan, 2001-2002.

Pastures

The established pastures are constituted by an association of Arachis pintoi with native grasses (AP+ GN) and occupy an area of 2.5 ha divided into seven sections and each of these into three subsections, in which intensive rotational grazing of 1 day of grazing and 20 days of recovery is carried out. The stocking rate applied during the experiment was 3.2 cows/ha during the rainy season (July-December) and 2 cows/ha the rest of the year.Prior to the establishment of Arachis pintoi, the herd grazed the native grass thoroughly; subsequently the legume was planted in the furrow at a depth of approximately 5 cm opened with a cultivator at a distance of 1 m. The vegetative material of Arachis pintoi came from stems selected in sections of 25 to 30 cm, planted between them in open vines every 0.5 m distance and 15 cm deep, leaving on the outside 1/3 of the length of each stem and the rest was covered with soil from the same vine, the first grazing occurred in May of (Castelán et al., 1998) and since then it has been grazed without interruption.

Variable s to be measured

The field evaluation began in March 2001 and was concluded in March 2002, i.e. a duration of 13 months. Samples for each variable were carried out according to Ibrahim (1994), as follows:

Flowering

Twelve estimations were made (one per month), beginning on March 3, 2001 and ending on March 23 of the following year. On each occasion, a metallic quadrant with dimensions of 0.0625 m^2 (0.25 x 0.25 m) was thrown at random fifty times, where the number of flowers present within the quadrant was counted, expressed as flowers/ha.

Seed reserve in the soil.

It was evaluated every 6 months, on three occasions: March 2001 (beginning), September and March 2002 (end). Fifty undisturbed cylindrical samples were taken (7.7 cm and 25 cm diameter and depth, respectively), from which the seed was recovered by washing and sieving, counting and weighing the seed. With this information the seed reserve was calculated, expressed as kg of seeds/ha and number of seeds/ha.

Seed quality and germination

From the seed recovered in March and September 2001, dark and light colored sub-samples were taken to determine the percentage of nitrogen, by means of the kjeldahl method (AOAC, 1980). The germination percentage was determined from the March 2002 collection, in three groups of 100 seeds each (light and/or dark), which were placed to germinate on moist blotting paper. The first group comprised seeds with dark (50) and light (50) coloration, assuming that the dark ones corresponded to mature seeds, while the light ones were considered to be still immature. The second group was only 100 light seeds. With this information, the unit seed weight, expressed in g/100 seeds, was also calculated.

Stolon density

In fifty quadrants of 0.0625 m^2 (0.25 x 0.25 m2), all stolons were cut, in which the total length was measured every 2 months in m/m^2 , as well as the number of rooting points (where one or more roots originate, regardless of size), which was expressed in points/m^2 .

Survival of plants and seedlings

In order to obtain a long-term estimate of adult seedling survival, in June 2001, seedlings were marked with plastic-coated wires. The plants were exposed to grazing (not isolated), and their survival was measured by direct observation. These observations were made every 7 days during the first month, every 14 days during the second month, successively extending the frequency of observation until the end of November of the same year. Plant survival was expressed as a percentage.

Statistical analysis

The collected data were subjected to analysis of variance to compare the measurements for each sampling month (except for plant survival and seed N and germination) to observe the trend of each variable (Steel and Torres, 1981), using the statistical package Genstat 5 (Agricultural Trust Lawes, 1996). The flowering and survival data were fitted to non-linear regression models to better visualize the time trend and to select those models that best predicted the information. For the case of flowering, the Gaussian peak equation was applied: $Y = y^0 + ae^{(0.5(x-x0/b)2)}$, where "Y" is the response variable (distribution of flowering) over time; y0 is the base value (left and right tails of the bell), and "ae" is the maximum value or cusp (peak). The exponential fraction$^{(-0.5\ (x-x0/b)2)}$, corresponding to the values that give the curve its "campaign" shape. For the case of "survival" the following exponential decay equation was used: $Y = Ae^{-bx}$, where "Y" is the percentage of survival at time "X" in days, "Ae" is the initial survival and "b" is the rate of disappearance of the plants.

RESULTS AND DISCUSSION

The presence of flowers in the evaluated plots showed an upward trend from the beginning of the observations (March 2001) until June of the same year.) Subsequently, a decline in the number of flowers was observed (March 2002). Figure 2 shows the behavior of this variable for all the plots. the experimental period. June 2001 showed the highest number of flowers (851 flowers m^2), and was statistically higher and different from the rest of the monthly observations (P≤0.001), while the minimum value was recorded in January 2002 with only 3 flowers/m^2. This last value was statistically similar to the averages of December 2001, February and March 2002. The average number of flowers/m^2 for the entire experimental period was 257± 268 flowers/m^2. The figure shows a greater variation in the presence of flowers during the summer months (June to September 2001).

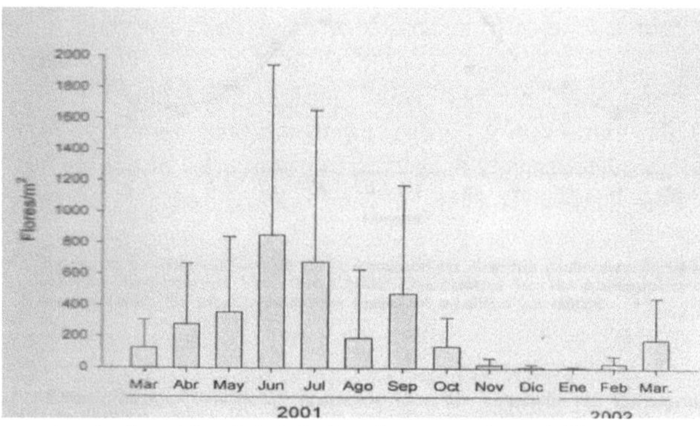

Figure 2. Flowering in Arachis pintoi during the experiment. Tlapacoyan, Ver. 2001-2002.The line above the bar is the standard error.

The figure shows that the lowest presence of flowers occurred during the "northern" or winter season, that is, when the ambient temperature in this region is lower than during the rest of the year.A non-linear Gaussian bell-shaped relationship was plotted with the available data, which indicated a normal distribution of flowering throughout the experimental period. The adjusted regression coefficient (R^2) was 0.70 (Figure3).

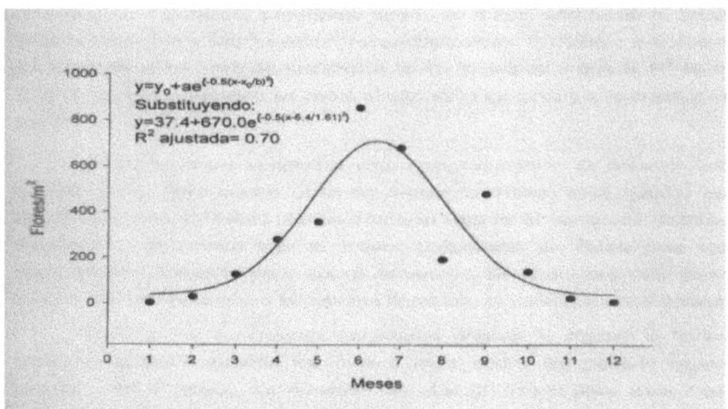

Figure3. Annual distribution of flowering in Arachis pintoi native grama association Tlapacoyan, Ver., 2001-2002. The dots are the actual observations. The Gauss equation was the best fit to the data.

This behavior coincides with a report by Enriquez (2001), who mentions that in Veracruz, Arachis pintoi does not flower during the "nortes" season due to the short photoperiod, high cloud cover and low temperatures.However, regarding flowering time, Castillo (2003), in this same experimental field, reported contrasting results for Arachis pintoi. Thus, in the first of the three years that were evaluated (1998, 1999 and 2000), the maximum average flowering occurred in September and November (minimum temperatures from 10° C to 15° C), with values of 54 and 119 flowers/m^2 , respectively. In the third year, the highest flowering was recorded in June and August (summer, maximum temperatures of 33° C and minimum temperatures of 19° C), with 573 flowers/m2. Additionally, this author pointed out that flowering maintained an important increase from the first to the third year, with values of 41, 98 and 346 flowers/m^2 , respectively. The model described in Figure 3 has a limited predictive value because R^2 is less than 0.85. It appears that this was due to the high value in June and the drastic drop in August.In temperate legumes, this seasonal flowering behavior also seems to occur, since in Argentina, Rosso et al. (2001) evaluated in 16 cultivars of white clover Trifolium repens the flowering distribution pattern and observed that the highest proportion of flowers for all ecotypes was found in the summer season. These authors reported that the cultivar churrinche recorded the highest flowering, averaging 530 flowers/m .^{2}

Drought conditions (Figure 1) also affect flowering, as was observed in the driest months of the experimental period (March, April and May). Arachis pintoi flowering for these months (on average) represented less than a third (28%) of the value recorded in June.In Paragominas, Brazil, Cruz et al., (1999) observed that the highest presence of Arachis pintoi flowers occurred in the rainiest month of the year (March) with 59 flowers/m^2 , while the lowest value occurred in the dry season (August). In temperate alfalfa (Medicago sativa) and fescue (Festuca arundinacea) grasslands,

Martín et. al., (2001) evaluated the association of these species to observe the effect of temperature and rainfall on plant population dynamics, in three planting seasons. They reported that the drought condition (high temperature and low humidity) affected seedling emergence of both species.

Seed reserves in the soil

The seed reserve observed in the soil showed some differences between the three correlations made (March and September 2001, and March 2002). Thus, the number of seeds per hectare for each collection was (rounded values) 15.8, 16.5 and 37.1 million seeds/ha, respectively. The weight per 100 seeds had a mean of 10.33 g in the three collections (Figure 4). From these data and considering the weight of 100 seeds, the yield in kg/ha was calculated, being for the first, second and third collection: 1671, 1388 and 3029 kg/ha, respectively (Figure 5). The analysis of variance showed that the number of seeds/ha of the first two collections were statistically equal but different from the third collection (P≤0.001). The average for the entire experimental period was 2029 kg/ha.Seed production in any crop is significantly affected mainly by environmental and soil fertility factors (Ferguson, 1995). In this regard, Enriquez (2001) evaluated, in the municipality of Isla, Ver., the effect of lime application from 0 to 3 tons/ha and harvest time (13, 15, and 17 months) on seed production in pods of Arachis pintoi CIAT 18744. The range of seed yield for all treatments was from 539 to 1703 kg/ha, but this author found no effect of lime dose applied, but only the effect of harvest age, with 1534, 1213, and 703 kg/ha, for 13, 15, and 17 months of age at harvest.In this same experimental field, Castillo (2002), evaluated the seed reserve of Arachis pintoi for the years 1998, 1999 and 2000. He reported 123, 207 and 764 kg/ha, respectively, which are lower than those mentioned here. In a clay oxisol soil of Paragominas, Brasil Cruz et al. (1999) evaluated in 1989 the seed production of Arachis pintoi. They applied 50 kg/ha of P2 O5, and harvested in March (rainy season (southern hemisphere) and August (dry season).

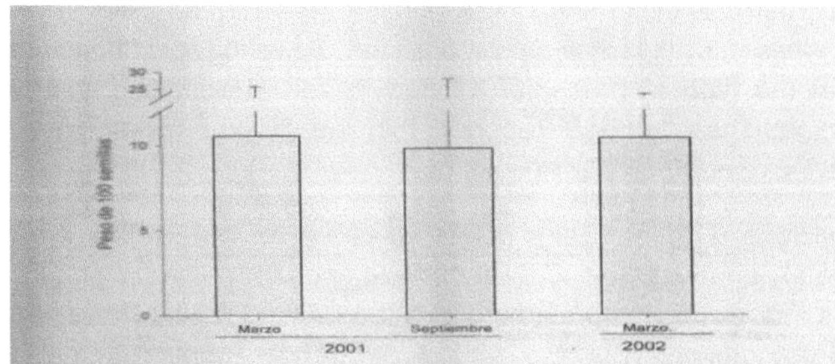

Figure 4. Weight of 100 arachis pintoi seeds associated with native grasses, in three samplings. Tlapacoyan, Ver., 2001.2002. The lines above the bars are the standard error.

In a literature review of arachis pintoi CIAT 18744 cultivar Porvenir, conducted by Angel and Villareal (1998), they reported that cultivar 17434 as the one evaluated in this work) produced, in Chinchina, Colombia, up to 7.28Ton/ha, 14 months after seed establishment, in soil of medium fertility and with good rainfall distribution, as opposed to seedlings established with vegetative material (stolons) and in more humid areas of Costa Rica, where they harvested between 800 and 2080 kg/ha. In all cases, cultivar 17434 produced more seed than cultivar Porvenir 18744.

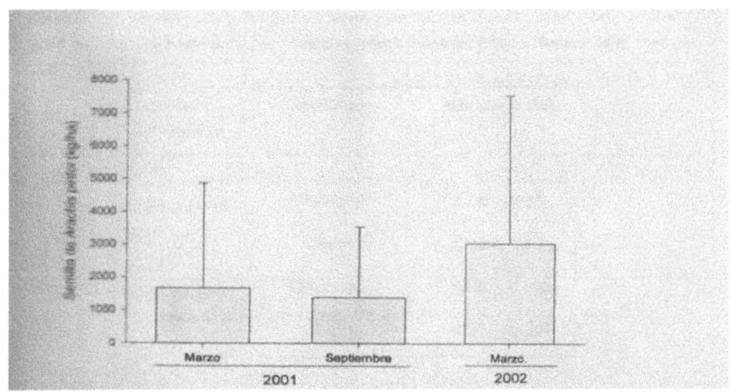

Figure 5. Arachis pintoi seed reserve associated with native grasses in the three samples. Tlapacoyan, Veracruz, 2001-2002. The lines above the bars are the standard error.

Seed quality and germination

Table 1 shows the information on the nitrogen content of Arachis pintoi seeds. It can be seen that the values of the March 2001 collection were (average of 3.7%) to those recorded in the September 2001 collection (6.0%). Regarding coloration, no trend was observed for this factor in relation to nitrogen content.

Table 1. Nitrogen content (%) in Arachis pintoi seed associated with native grasses, collected in March and September 2001, 2001. Tlapacoyan, Ver. 2001-2002.

Seed collected in	Coloring	Nitrogen (%)
March 2001	Obscure	4.5 0 ±.38
	Claras	3.36 ± 0.53
September 2001	Obscure	5.93 ± 0.23
	Claras	6.13 ± 0.36

The germination percentage of the seeds collected in March 2002 averaged 43.7% for all cases (3 samples, and dark and light seed color). Table 2 presents in detail the percentages achieved for each of the three samples evaluated and their respective color. In this case, it appears that the dark color (mature seeds) was decisive in achieving higher germination (average 50%) compared to light or immature seeds (15.5%).

Table 2. Seed germination percentage of Arachis pintoi associated with native grasses. Tlapacoyan, Ver. 2001- 2002.

Number of germinated seeds				
Group of 100 seeds	Coloring	Obscure	Claras	Percentage of germination
1	Obscura and clear			
	Obscure		-----------	
	Claras			

Stolon density

The values of stolon density/m^2 in Arachis ppintoi plants showed at the first estimates, a trend The first estimates show a downward trend corresponding to the period March-July 2001, and then rebounded from September of the same year until March of the following year (Figure 6). The estimates estimates made at March of 2001-2002 presented the The analysis of variance showed significant differences (P ± 0.001) between the averages, with the March 2001 and 2002 samples being the same and the July 2001 samples being the lowest. The analysis of variance showed significantly significant differences (P ± 0.001) between the averages, with the March 2001 and 2002 samples being equal and higher than the March 2002 samples. That the rest.

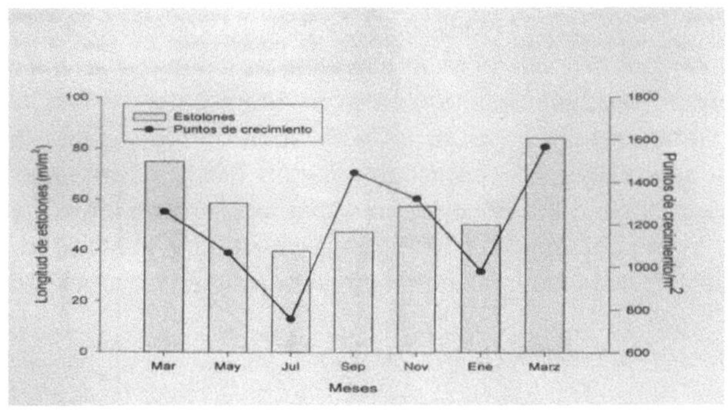

Stolon length and growing points in Arachis pintoi associated with native grama. Tlapacoyan, ver., 2001-2002.

Survival of plants and seedlings

Survival was strongly affected during the first 15 days of life. Thus, by that date (16/06/2001) almost half of the initially emerged seedlings had already disappeared. Subsequently, until the end of the observations on day 166 (11/11/2001), the rate of disappearance stabilized with an average percentage (per observation) of 5.5%, leaving 6.5% at the end of the observation period. plants out of the 120 originally marked. The initial abrupt drop in seedling survival is shown in Fig. 7, where the actual observations/points) were plotted with an exponential decay equation, where "Y" is the percent initial survival (100%), "b" is the rate of plant disappearance, and "x" is the time in days. The regression coefficient was high (R^2 =0.9).

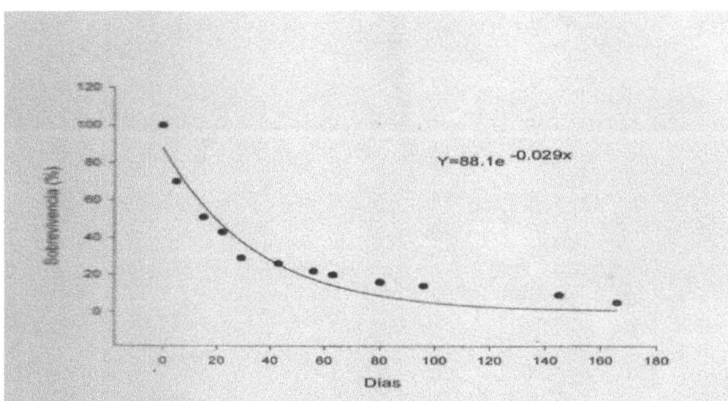

Survival percentage of Arachis pintoi plants originally planted during the period June-November 2001. Tlapacoyan, Ver., 2001- 2002. Dots are actual observations.

23

Although Argel and Villarreal (1998) mention that the persistence of Arachis pintoi relies on the abundant biomass of seed and stolons, it seems that this persistence is based more on its propagation through stolons (from other stolons or true seeds), than through viable seeds, because as was seen in the results, the survival of seedlings from seeds was low, particularly during the first two weeks of life. This reasoning is strengthened if it is considered that when rooting, the stolons "assure" their presence in the soil, besides being physically better adapted to compete and resist adverse conditions in the pasture, mainly due to pests, diseases or trampling.

CONCLUSIONS

1. It would seem that flowering depended more on environmental temperature than on soil moisture availability; thus, minimum temperatures during the winter season (even with high rainfall) significantly depressed flowering of Arachis pintoi, putting the survival of the species at risk.

2. The possibility of creating an important seed reserve in the soil that guarantees the persistence of the species in the pasture increased as time went by. This is confirmed by other local experiences with Arachis pintoi.

3. The drier months of the experimental period favored the length of stolons in the field, thus benefiting the survival of the species during the critical period. A similar behavior was observed for the growing points.

4. The quantity of seeds and stolons in the field was the determining factor for the survival of the species, since the persistence of individual plants was poor over time.

LITERATURE CITED

Agriculture trust laws.1996. Genstat 5" second edition, reread 3.2 ed.agricultural, IACR, Rthamsed, UK.

AOAC. 1980. Official Methods of Analysis 13th ed Asociation of Official Analytical Chemists. Washington, D.C.

Argel, P.J. and M. Villarreal. 1998. New Perennial Forage Peanut (Arachis pintoi Krapovickas and Gregory). Cultivar Porvenir (CIAT 18744).BOLETINJ TECCNICO Ministerio de Agricultura de Costa Rica (MAG), Centro Internacional de Agricultura Tropical (CIAT). Technical Bulletin. 32 P.

Arzola, A; Castillo, E; Valles B; Jarillo, J. 1997. No-tillage establishment of Arachisnpintoi and Phaseloides puerperia in native pastures. Tropical Pastures (19) 3:51-54.

Azakawa, N.M. and C.A.R. Ramirez. 1989. Methodology for inoiculation and masting of Arachis pintoi. PasturasTropicales 11 (1): 24-26.

Bosman, H:G:; E. Castillo, B. Valles and Lucia (de), G.R. 1990. Botanical composition and noduation of legumes in native pastures of the coastal plain of the Gulf of Mexico. Pasturas Tropicales 12 (1): 2-8.

Cadisch, G:R:M. Schunke and K. E. Giller (1994). Nitrogen cycling in a pure grass pasture and a grass-legume mixture on a red latozol in Brazil. 1999.

Castelan, R:G., G. E. Castillo, L.t Mannetje, B. Valles, A. Aluja and M. Torres. 1998. Production and botanical composition of three Arachis pintoi accessions associated with a native grassland of the humid tropics of the state of Veracruz, during the year of establishment. 13-15. In CEIEGT Newsletter 1997. Centro de Enseñanza e Investigación y Extensión en Ganadería Tropical, FMVZ-UNAM. Martínez de la Torre, Ver.

Castillo, G.E. 2000. Milk production in native pastures associated with legume Arachis pintoi. In Proceedings of the Course: Milk Production and

(E. Castillo and J. Jarillo, Eds). Centro de Enseñanza e Investigación y Extensión en Ganadería Tropical, FMVZ- UNAM. Martínez de la Torre, Ver 86 p.

Castillo, G. E. 2003. Improving a native Pasture with The legume Arachis pintoi in the Himididid Tropics of Mexico. Ph.D. Thesis Wageningen University. The Netherlands. 157 p.

Chantal, V. 1998. Quality ad quantity of forage from a native pasture alonenornAassociated with Arachis pintoi CIAT 17434 (no page numbers). Agricultural University of Wageningen . The Netherland.

CATIE (Tropical Agricultural Research and Higher Education Center) 1990. Evaluation of star grass (Cynodon nlemfuensis) alone and associated with forage legumes Arachis pintoi CIAT and Desmodium ovalifolium CIAT 350 on milk production and its components: First annual report (MAG/IDA/CATIE/CIID) Turrialba, Costa Rica. P 104-120.

CIAT (International Center for Tropical Agriculture). 1990 Tropical Forage Programs. Annual Report 1990. Working Papers No. 89. Cali, Colombia. P 911.

CIAT. (International Center for Tropical Agriculture). 1997 Tropical Grasses and Legumes. 86-87. Optimization of Genetic Diversity for Multiple Uses (IP-5 Projects) CIAT): Annual Report 1996. Cali, Colombia.

Cook, B.G., R.J. Williams, And G.P.M. Wilson (1990). Archis pintoi Krap. Et Greg. Nom. Nud. (pinto peanut) cv. Amarillo. Australian Journal of Experimental Agriculture 30: 445-446.

Cruz, E. D., M. Simao e J.L. Covre. 1999. Seed production of Arachis pintoi Krap. Et. Grep. Na Amazonia Oriental Brasileira. Pasturas Tropicales 21 (3): 59-61.

Enriquez, Q.F.J. and G. E. Castillo. 1996. Recently introduced pastures in the tropics of Mexico. Course on milk production in tropical climates. March 18-22. <<Instituto Tecnológico No. 4 SEP-SEIT-DGETA. Altamira, Tamaulipas, Mexico.

Enriquez, Q.F.J. 2001. Effect of lime application and harvest time on seed production of Arachis pintoi CIAT 18744. Tropical Pastures 23(1):25-28.

Ferguson, J.E. 1995. Seed biology and seed production systems for arachis pintoi 131-143 In: Biology and Agronomy of Arachis pintoi Forage Species (P.C. kerridge, ed). International Center for Tropical Agriculture (CIAT). Cali, Colombia. Publication No. 245.

Fisher. M.J and P. Cruz. 1995. Some ecophysiology of Arachis pintoi . 56-75. In: Biology and agronomy of Arachis pintoi forage species (P:C kerridge, ed). International Center for Tropical Agriculture (ciat). Cali, Colombia. Publication No. 245,

Guardener, C.J. 1982. Pupulation dynamics and stability of stylosanthes hamata Cv. Verano in grazed pastures. Australian Journal of Agricultural Research 33(1): 63-74.

Giller, K.E., And K.F. Wilson. 1991. Nitrogen Fixation in Tropipical, Cropping System CAB International , Wallingford UK.

Gómez-Cortéz, G.E., B, Valles. Castillo and J. Jarillo 1994. Evaluation of methods for the establishment of Arachis pintoi in a pasture in Veracruz, Mexico. Pasturas Tropicales Pasturas Tropicales 16(1): 15-21.
Grof, B. (1985) Forage Attributes of the perennial groundnut Arachis pintoi in a tropical savanna environment in Colombia. In International Grassland Congress, pp.

67-85, Japan.

Harris W. 1978.Defolation as a determinant of the growth, persistence and composition of pasture. 67-85 I: John, R. W. (ed). Plant relation in pastures. CSIRO, Merbourne Australia.

Harper, J.L. 1977. Population Biology of plants. Academic Press, London. 892 p.
Harper, J.L. 1978 relation in pastures. 3-14 In: Plant relations in pastures: (willson

R. J. ed). CSIRO, Melbourne Australia.
Hernández, T., B. Valles y E. Castillo. 1990: Evaluation of forage grasses and legumes in Veracruz. Pasturas Tropicales (12) 3:29-33.

Hernández M., P. J. Argel, M.A. Ibrahim and L. mannejet. 1995. Pasture production, diet selection an liveweight gains of cattle grazing Brachiaria brizantha with or without Arachis pintoi at 2 stocking rate in the Atlantic zone of Costa Rica. Tropical grasslands (29) 3: 134-141.

Hodgkinson, K.C. and O.B. Williams, 1983. Adaptation of grazing in forage plants. 85-100. In Genetic resources of plants (McIvor, J.G. And Bray, R. A. Eds). CSIRO, Melbourne, Australia.

Humphreys, LR.   1981.Environmental adapatation of tropical pasture plants.

Mc.Millan Publishers Ltd., London. 261 p.
Humphreys, LR. 1991. Tropical Pasture utilization. Cambridge University press.

Melbourne, Australian 206 p.
Hibrahim, M.A. 1994. Compatibility, Persistence and Productivity of grass-legume Mixtures for Sustainable Animal Production in the atlantic Zone of Costa Rica (Ph.D. Thesis) Wagenningen, The Netherlands. Department of Agronomy. Wageningen Agriculture University. 129.9.

Hibrahim, M.A. and L. Mannetge 1998. Compatibility, persistence and productivity of grass-legume mixture in the humid tropics of Costa Rica. 1. Dry matter yied, nitrogen yield and botanical composition. Tropical Grasslands 32(2): 96,104.

Jones, R: M: 1982. White clover (Trifolium repens) in subtropical south-east Queensland. I Some Effects of site, Season an management practices on the population dynamics of White clover. Tropical Grasslands 16(3): 118-127.

Jones, R: M G.A. Bunch. 1988. The effect of stoking rateo n the population dinamycs of Siratro in Siratro (Macroptilium atropurpurium) Setaria (Settaria sphacelata) pastures in southeast Queesland; 1: Survival of Plants and Stolons. Aust. J. Agric. Res. 39(2): 209-219.

Jones, R: M and "t "L. Mannetje. 1986. A. comparison of bred Macroptilium lines and cv. Siratro in subcoastal southeast with special reference to legume persistence. Commonwealth Scientific and industrial Research Organisation (CSIRO), Div. Trop.

Crops and Pastures, Trop. Agr. Tech. Memo: no. 47.11 p.

Jones, R: M and E. D. Carter. 1989. Demography of pasture legume. 139-158. In: Persistence of Forrage Lugemes (Marten, G.C. Ed.) American Society Of Agronomy Inc. Madison, Wisconsin, USA.

Lascano, C.E. and P.C. Avila. 1991. Milk production potential in pastures alone and associated with legumes adapted to acid soils. Pasturas tropicales 12(3): 2-10.

Manenetje 't, L.S.J. Cook and J.H. Wildin. 1983. The effects of fire on buffel grass with Siratro pasture. Tropical Grassland 17:30-39.

Manenetje 't, L. 1989.Productivity and persistence of legumes and their adoption in tropical pastures. >In: Proceedings of a Workshop. Contribution of improved pastures to animal production in the tropics. CIAT International Center for Tropical Agriculture. Cali, Colombia. P 25-38.

Manenetje 't, L. 1995. Long-term effects of stocking rate and management on population dynamics of grazing forage legume plants 1-.
12. In memoirs of the course on biological basis of high density grazing.

(G..E. Castillo, Editor) de Investigación, Enseñanza y Extensión en Ganadería Tropical, Facultad de Medicina Veterinaria y Zootecnia, UNAM. Martinez de la Torre, Veracruz

Manenetje 't, L. 1995b. Practical technologies for improving pastures in Central America. 13-22. In Proceedings of the course: Biological basis of high density grazing (E.G. Castillo, Editor). Centro de Investigación, Enseñanza, Enseñanza y Extensión en Ganadería Tropical, Facultad de Medicina Veterinaria y Zootecnia, UNAM. Martínez de la Torre, Ver.

Martin B.R. Refi., S Montico and M. Constanzo. 2001. Effect of climatic factor on the plant population dynamics in temperature implantation (ID#01-12). XIX International Grassland congress. 11-21 February, 2001. Sao Paulo, Brazil

Mckeon, G.M. And J. J. Mott. 1984 Agronomy Seed Biology of Stylosanthes. 311-355. In The Biology and Agronomy os stylosanthes. (Stance, H.M. And L.A. EDye. Eds.) Academic Press, Syndney, Australia.

McWilliam, J.R. 1978. Response of pastures plants to temperature. 17-34 In: Plan Relations in pastures (Wilson, R.J. ed). SCIRO, Melbourne. Australia.

Mire, R. M. 1991. Pasture management for fattening. 2-16. In: Balance Alimentario de Bovinos (Ruiz, R., Guerrero, M.A., Galina, H. y Ruíz, C. eds.) Facultad de Estudios Superiores (FES) Cuautitlán UNAM. Mexico. MEXICO CITY.

Minson, D. 1990. Forrage in Ruminat nutrition. San Diego. Academic. Press 483 p.

Monsalve, L. R. 200. Botanical composition of forage ingested by F1 cows (Holsteins) grazing native grama and native grama associated with Arachis pintoi, during the transition between rainy and northerly seasons in a site with Af(m) climate in the state of Veraruz Mexico. Bachelor's thesis, Faculty of Veterinary Medicine, Universidad de Ciencias Aplicadas y Ambientales, Bogotá, Colombia; and Faculty of Veterinary Medicine and Zootechnics, Universidad Nacional Autónoma de México. 54 p.

Pizarro, E.A., M. A. Carvalho, and A.K. B. Ramos. 1998, Effect of cutting frequency on seed production of Araachis pintoi. Pasturas Tropicales 20 (1):31-33.

Ramos, V.A. 1983. Bovine production systems in four municipalities of the state of Veracruz. Licentiate thesis. UNAM, Mexico.

Rincón, C.A. 1994. Production potential of Arachis pintoi ecotypes in the Piedemonte of the Eastern Plains of Colombia. Pasturas Tropicales 23. (1): 19-21.

Rincón, C.A. and Argulles, M.G. 1991 Perennial forage peanut (Arachis pintpoi) Krapovickas and Gregory): An Alternative for the Agricultural Sector Ministry of Agriculture of Colombia, Colombian Agricultural Institute (ICA), International Center for Tropical Agriculture (CIAT). 18 p.

Rasso, B.>s. E.M. Pagano, And P. Remero. 2001. Flowering distribution pottem in White clover cultivar (ID 03-03). XIX International Grasslands Congress. 11- 21 11-21 February, 2001, Sao Paulo, Brazil.

Rosisiter, R.C. 1978. The ecology of subterranean clover-based pasture 325- 339.In: Plant Relations in Pastures (Wilson R.J. ed). CSIRO, Melbourne. Australia.

Valls, J:F; Simpson. C.E. 1993. Taxonomy Natural Distribution, and Attributes of Arachis pintoi 1-18. In<. Kerridge, P.C., and B. Hardy (eds). Biology and agronomic of forage Arachis p. International Center for Tropical Agriculture (CIAT). Cali Colombia.

Van Heurck, L.M. 1990. Evaluation of Estrella grass (Cynodon nlemfuensis) alone and associated with the forage legumes Arachis pintoi CIAT 17434 and Desmodium ovalifolium CIAT 350 on milk production and its components (Master's thesis). Turrialva, Costa Rica. Tropical Agricultural Research and Higher Education Center (CATIE). 152 p.

Villarreal M., and L. Zúñiga. 1996. Frequency of cutting production of Arachis pintoi accessions. 45-49 In: P.J. Argel and A. Ramírez, eds. Regional experience with Arachos pintoi and future plans for research and promotion of the species in Mexico, Central America and the Caribbean. International Center for Tropical Agriculture (CIAT), Cali. Colombia.

CHAPTER II

Ingestive behavior of cows in a native grass/Arachis pintoi association.
in the humid tropics of Veracruz
Epigmenio Castillo Gallegos, Rodrigo Rascón Chincoya, Diana García
González, Jesús Jarillo Rodríguez, Andrés Aluja Schunemann, Len 't Manne.

INTRODUCTION

Native grasses constitute between 25 and 75 % of the pastures in the Mexican humid tropics dedicated to cattle breeding and dual purpose livestock. These pastures are not very productive due to low soil fertility. Arachis pintoi (Ap) is a persistent legume, effective N fixer[2] , which is adapted to warm and humid conditions. Therefore, it was proposed that the best way to improve the sustainable production of native grasses (NG) would be the introduction of A. pintoi. Three and a half years after its introduction, the soil of the grass with legume (GN+Ap) showed slightly higher carbon levels than the control pasture of native grass.The initial value of carbon at 20 cm depth in 1998 was 24.7 t/ha and the average increase until 2001 was 3.7 t/ha/yr and 4.8 t/ha/yr for NG and NG+Ap, respectively. The GN+Ap treatment added to the soil 60 kg/ha/year of N. Soil bulk density was not affected by the treatments, being its mean of 1.21 g/ cm3. In conclusion, the increases in C and N due to the introduction of Arachis. pintoi in native grasses could constitute an environmental bonus for pasture agroecosystems in the Mexican humid tropics.DM intake, as well as its quality and relationship with ruminant feeding behavior, has been studied in pastures associated with introduced grasses and Arachis pintoi with mainly meat-producing breeds (4, 5, 6). However, these studies are scarce in associations of native grasses with Arachis pintoi and with other types of animals, which are necessary because native grasses are an induced vegetation of great importance in the Depending on the region, they make up 25 to 70 % of the grazing areas (7). Native grasses produce less biomass and lower quality biomass than introduced grasses.Native grasses produce less biomass and lower quality biomass than introduced grasses. In addition, their growth is markedly seasonal, but their establishment is simple and inexpensive, and once established they are persistent (7).DM intake, as well as its quality and the relationship with ruminant feeding behavior, has been studied in pastures associated with introduced grasses and Arachis. pintoi with mainly meat-producing breeds (4, 5, 6). pintoi and with other types of animals, which are necessary because native grasses are an induced vegetation of great importance in dual purpose cattle raising in the Mexican tropics, since depending on the region, they form from 25 to 70 % of the grazing areas (7). Native grasses produce less biomass, and this is of lower quality, than introduced grasses. In addition, their growth is markedly seasonal, but their establishment is simple and inexpensive, and once established they are persistent (7). ....

The grazing feeding of the animal while grazing, understood as the activities and time that each activity takes the animal to acquire the food that nourishes it. Such activities are: grazing, ruminating, and other di st i nta l activities, such as drinking water, walking and resting, either lying or standing. Through direct observations it is possible to quantify the time taken by the animal for each activity. For this reason, it is also advisable to describe the animal's feeding behavior and how it is affected by pasture management (2). In addition, the quantity and quality of dry matter (DM) ingested are necessary measurements to explain differences in animal production of pastures whose administration is different (3). DM intake, as well as its quality and relationship with ruminant feeding behavior, has been studied in pastures associated with introduced grasses and Arachis pintoi with mainly meat-producing breeds (4, 5, 6). However, this iss es tud ies son esca sos en associationsof native grasses with Arachis. Pintoiand withother types of animals, and which are necessary because native grasses are an induced vegetation of great importance in dual purpose cattle raising in the Mexican tropics, since depending on the region concerned, they form from 25 to 70% of the grazing areas(7).

Target

The objective of this study was to determine the effect of introducing Arachis pintoi CIAT 17434 into a native grass pasture on the quality of forage intake and grazing behavior of dual-purpose cows (F1, Holstein x Cebu) in the humid tropics of the state of Veracruz.

MATERIAL AND METHODS

The study was carried out during the rainy season, from June 25 to August 14, 2000, at the Centro de Enseñanza, Investigación y Extensión en Ganadería Tropical (CEIEGT) of the Facultad de Medicina Veterinaria y Zootecnia of the UNAM, which is located about 40 km west of the Gulf of Mexico coastline (20° 02' N, 97° 06' W , 112 masl). There are three climatic seasons: rainy (July-October), with high rainfall and temperatures; winter or "nortes" (November-February), with low temperatures and less rainfall than the previous one; and dry (March-June) with high temperatures and little rainfall. The nortes and drought are periods of low grass growth due to low temperatures and high evaporative demand, respectively. The soils are acid ultisols (pH 5.4), with low phosphorus (1- 2 ppm; Bray II) and nitrogen (0.0018 %) contents and average organic matter contents (2.4 %); their texture is silty clay. The thin arable layer (0 to 25 cm) rests directly on the soil. The native grasses used in this study originated from pastures of introduced species that were established at the beginning of the 1980s, and then were gradually invaded by the native grasses ([6]. The native grass (NP) pastures used in the present study originated from pastures of introduced species that were established at the beginning of the 1980s, and then were gradually invaded, mainly by native grasses and some l e gumineae, which became dominant at the beginning of the 1990s. Among the native grasses present in significant quantities are the braid grasses (Paspalum notatum and Paspalum. plicatulum), folder (Axonopus affinis and A. compressus), foxtail (Setaria sp), Bermuda (Cynodon dactylon) and important weeds such as the grasses a (Paspalum virgatum) and savanna (Sporobolus poiretii). Although with lesser content in the botanical composition, there are the leguminous pega-pega (Desmodium spp) and others considered as weeds, such as the pinahuistle (Mimosa pigra).

Pasture management

These pastures received rotational grazing (2 to 3 days of grazing, 50 to 70 days of recovery) with an average stocking rate of 1.25 AU/ha between December 1993 and October 1994, period in which their botanical composition was: 39 % of introduced grasses (GI), 48 % of native grasses (GN), 3 % of broadleaf weeds (MA), 6 % of narrowleaf weeds (MN) and 5 % of native legumes (LN).There were two treatments: the native grass pasture (PN) as a control and the experimental pasture (PNA), in which Arachis pintoi (CIAT 17434) was introduced; each occupied 2.5 ha. The first was implemented in 1996 from already established native grasses. Arachis. pintoi was planted vegetatively in the native grasses using an inter-row spacing of 1.0 m and 0.5 m between plants, between August and November 1996, and was grazed for the first time in May 1997.Each pasture was divided into 21 paddocks in order to carry out the rotational grazing of 1 day of grazing for 20 days of rest. The stocking rate applied during the experimental period was 3.2 cows/ha, which according to the weights of the cows, was cows during the experiment were equivalent to 3.2 and 3.6 animal units (AU= 450 kg BW) per hectare for NP and NAP, respectively. Eight intact cows (VIN, without esophageal fistula), F1 cross (Holstein x Zebu) per treatment, whose average weight ± standard deviation was 450 ± 64 kg for PN and 505 ± 61 kg for PNA, were managed in a dual-purpose system, with milking once a day in the morning, during which time they were supplemented with approximately 1.2 kg molasses/cow/day (" 1 kg DM/cow/day). In their first four months of lactation they nursed their calves for 30 min after milking (08:00 h) and for the same time in the afternoon (14:00 h). Two fistulated esophageal fistulated cows (FEV), of the ¾ Holstein - ¼ zebu crossbreed, which grazed similar paddocks to the experimental ones and weighed on average 576 ± 68 kg, were also used.Additionally, there were three bulls with ruminal fistula provided with permanent cannulas with removable plugs, whose average weight was 550 ± 65 kg. Measurements on the pastures and animals were carried out from June 25 to August 14, 2000. To avoid causing stress to the cows fistulated to the esophagus due to frequent sampling, measurements of ingestive behavior were made first in the NAP treatment, during the 21 consecutive days of the grazing cycle (period 1, June 25 to July 15) and then, in the NP treatment in the following cycle (period 2, July 25 to August 14). 21 paddocks of each treatment were sampled, estimating the DM present (DM, kg/ha) before grazing with the comparative yield method(8).

Forage sampling

In the reference quadrats, forage was cut at ground level and then dried in forced air oven for 48 h at 62 °C to estimate DM content .Botanical composition (BC, %) was estimated with the dry weight rank method (9). Dry matter present (DM) and botanical composition (BC) were visually graded in 100 quadrats per paddock. Botanical components were considered: Arachis. pintoi (AP), native grasses (GN) and introduced grasses (GI), broadleaf (MA) and narrowleaf (MN) weeds and native legumes (LN). Likewise, in the botanical composition (BC), bitter grass (Paspalum virgatum) and savanna (Sporobolus poiretii) were considered as individual species and not within the group of native grass species, since they are important weeds in the experimental pastures and at the regional level, besides being little consumed by cattle. The main species in the different botanical groups were: native grasses: bahiagrass (Paspalum notatum), Paspalum dilatatatum, Paspalum plicatulum, Paspalum conjugatum, carpet grasses (Axonopus affinis and Axonopus compressus), Bermuda grass (Cynodon dactylon) and Setaria spp.Introduced grasses: African star grass (Cynodon plectostachius), Sunday star grass (Cynodon nlenfuensis) and tanner grass (Brachiaria arrecta); narrow-leaved weeds: Cyperus spp.; broad-leaved weeds: Ecobilla (Sida acuta) and leguminous plants: Dormilona (Mimosa pudica) and Pinahustle (Mimosa. Pigra); and native leguminous plants: - Desmodium, Rhynchosia and Centrosema species. The botanical components considered in the esophageal extrusion were: Arachis pintoi, native legumes, grasses and other species. A sub-sample of 400 g of fresh extrudate was taken and spread evenly on a tray, which was examined. The botanical composition of the extrusa was calculated from 400 points observed under the stereoscopic microscope along the length of the tray. This technique is a modification of that employed by Harker et al (10). Grazing feeding behavior was measured by direct observation of grazing activities, either visually, auditorily, or both at the same time (2). These measurements were made every other day and every other day, so seven measurements were made during the 21-day grazing cycle.

Cow grazing behavior

In the first grazing cycle, feeding behavior was measured in the eight cows that grazed the associated pasture, and in the second period, in the other eight cows that were on native grasses alone. The activity of the intact cows was classified as: grazing or grazing (TP, min/24 h), when the animal was visually observed with its head down, close to the ground, pinning or about to graze a portion of the pasture; rumination (TR, min/24 h), when the cow was ruminating either standing or lying down; and other activities (TO, min/24 h), if the animal was neither grazing nor ruminating and was standing, lying down or walking.
These variables were recorded on each animal at 10-min intervals for 24 continuous hours, starting at 15:00 h. The total time per activity was the product of the number of records per 10 min, assuming that each record represented activity in the subsequent 10 min. The total time per activity was the product of the number of records per 10 min, assuming that each record represented the activity in the subsequent 10 min. Ten seconds were used to confirm the recorded activity.

Bite rate

Bite rate (TB, bites/min) and bite size (TM, g MO/bite) were estimated using the two cows fistulated to the esophagus, which were allowed to graze for 30 to 40 min in the morning and afternoon, during which time bites were counted in the effective grazing time, usually 30 min. TB was equal to the number of bites recorded divided by the effective grazing time. The bite was defined as the characteristic sound produced when the grass is separated from the pasture by the cow, which is easily audible (11). The TM was calculated by dividing the weight of organic matter (OM) of esophageal extrusion collected by the total number of bites, both variables recorded during the effective grazing time. Dry matter (DM), organic matter (OM) and crude protein (CP) contents were determined in the esophageal extrusion (12). Although the information generated from the extrusion does not allow us to accurately assess the quality of the diet, it does allow us to generate values that indicate differences between diets that can explain the productive results.

Method for measuring dry matter consumption

To measure dry matter intake, chromium dioxide ($Cr_2 O_3$) was used as an external marker to estimate daily excreta production. Intact cows were dosed daily for 21 days with exactly 4 g/day of the tracer.The first 14 days were considered necessary to achieve the state of continuous and uniform flow of the tracer along the gastrointestinal tract; fecal samples were collected individually directly from the rectum of each animal in the last seven days. A composite stool sample was formed from daily aliquots, and Cr content was determined by atomic absorption spectroscopy (13).

Excrement production

Excrement production was obtained with the formula: [(g of Cr dosed)*(Recovery rate)] / [Cr] in excreta; a recovery rate of 82.5 %, based on the information presented by Danes et al (14) The DM digestibility of the ingested grass (extrudate) was estimated with the in situ method after 48 h of ruminal incubation (15) samples of esophageal extrudate, which were introduced already dried and ground with a (Wiley Mill # 4, 1 mm sieve) in triplicate to the rumen; those animals besides the grass that they consumed freely in a paddock of 6.6 ha pasture, consisting mainly of Tanner (Brachiaria arrecta), Star (Cynodon nlemfuensis) and native grasses (Paspalum spp, Axonopus spp) received from five days before, until the end of all runs, 2 kg of feed concentrate (16% CP, 88% DM) per animal per day, in order to ensure a uniform microbial population in number and activity; The commercial bags used were made of white polyester monofilament fabric with a pore size of 53 ± 10 microns and are nitrogen-free, with a size of 10 cm x 20 cm.

Dry matter (DM) consumption

Organic matter intake (CMO, kg/cow/day) was calculated as follows (13): Fecal production (g OM/cow/day)/ 1 - organic matter (OM) digestibility. Saleable milk production (PLV, kg/cow/day) was recorded daily during the two 21-day grazing cycles that lasted the experiment (42 days in total); 15 of the 16 cows were lactating and of these, six were raising their calf, two on native pasture (NP) and four on native pasture plus Arachis pintoi (ANP). Each week, calves were weighed before and after suckling to obtain, by difference, the daily calf milk intake (CLB, kg/day). Total milk production (PLT, kg/cow/day) was the sum of PLV + CLB, and in case the cow had no calf, PLV was equal to PLT. The response variables measured in the pasture and in the animals had as replicates the paddock and the animals, respectively.

Variance analysis

The analysis of variance was performed with the PROC GLM procedure of SAS (16). In the case of the analysis of variance of milk production, the number of days in lactation at the beginning of the experiment and the number of calving, as well as the measurement period, were used as covariates. In all cases, the level of statistical significance used was P<0.05.In both measurement periods, the minimum and maximum temperatures did not differ greatly from the historical averages. However, in period 1 it rained a quarter of the historical average, while in period 2 it rained 23 mm more than the historical average. The associated pasture had significantly 27 % more MSP before grazing than the control.

Contribution of botanical composition in grassland

The contribution of Arachis pintoi to the botanical composition was approximately 28 %. The contributions of native grasses, introduced grasses and savanna grass were significantly higher in the control than in the association. Also, the control had significantly 1.5 times more broadleaf weeds than the PNA treatment.The contribution of bittergrass and native legumes was statistically equal in both treatments (Table 2). The percentage of Arachis. pintoi in the esophageal extrusion was 1.5 times more than that of the pasture. (Table 2), 3), while the amount of grasses in NP was significantly higher than that of ANP. The content of native legumes and other species in the esophageal extrusion, being very low, was not a determining factor in DM intake or diet quality.Crude protein and in situ digestibility of OM of the esophageal extrudate were significantly higher in ANP than in NP (Table 3). Both the linear and quadratic effects of the percentage of A. pintoi in the extrudate were significant on in situ digestibility of MO and CP and (Figure 1), the respective equations being :DISMO= 29.40 + 1.14*PCTAP - 0.0129*PCTAP2, R2= 0.25, n = 28; (P<0.05)PC= 3.35 + 0.53*PCTAP -0.0056*PCTAP2, R2=0.39, n= 28; (P<0.05) Grazing time was statistically similar in both treatments, while rumination time was significantly lower in ANP than in NP. The difference in time spent in other activities was significant in favor of ANP. Bite rate of PN was significantly higher than that of PNA, with the opposite occurring with bite size.The consumption of OM by the double marker method was similar among treatments (Table 3). On the other hand, OM consumption calculated from ingestive behavior resulted in lower graphical values, with the control treatment showing a significantly higher consumption than the association.Saleable milk production and calf milk consumption were statistically equal among treatments. However, total milk production per cow from the associated pasture significantly exceeded that of the control (Figure 2). In a grazing experiment, MSP has little value by itself. It is more rational to express MSP in terms of availability: units of forage offered per units of animal live weight, as this can be related to both intake and productive performance per animal (17). In tropical pastures, the availability to reach maximum production per animal is variable, from 5 to 35 kg DM/100 kg BW; this wide range is due to differences among experiments with respect to pasture type, nutritional quality and management, which makes it difficult to apply the results of an experiment to particular situations.The grazing ruminant ingests leaves and very little stem, so it would be reasonable to express availability as DM-green (18) or better, in terms of leaf DM-green. In the present case, the content of senescent material was practically nil, so that availability, although not expressed as such, was mainly DM-green. Likewise, during the study, the average availability was 10.9 and 12.2 kg DM/100 kg DM in the control and associated pastures, respectively, which falls within the wide range mentioned above. In addition, the average availability was 5.0 and 5.8 times the dry matter intake estimated by $Cr_2 O_3$ -digestibility in situ (Table 3).The MSP utilization rates of the present experiment were 14.0 and 11.5 % for PN and PNA, respectively. Previously, Monsalve et al (19) estimated utilization rates of 11.4 and 13.6 % for the same treatments, values that are in general agreement with the literature, which indicates low levels of utilization for tropical pastures, between 10 and 40 % (19).Dry matter present (DM) alone can influence milk intake and milk production. Cowan and O' Grady (20) showed that milk production per cow was constant when DM>2,500 kg/ha, but that below 2,000 kg both intake and grazing time were reduced. Therefore, in the present experiment, cows in both treatments were not exposed to deficit levels of PSM that limited voluntary intake (Table 2). MSP quality was sufficiently high so as not to present limits to forage intake. CP values were in all cases above the critical range of 6 to 8 % below which N deficiency for ruminal microbes is more likely and could reduce intake. Likewise, OM digestibility values were at the high end of the range for tropical pastures, with or without legumes, as cited by Minson (3).This is in agreement with other results (21) for the nutritive value of samples obtained by manually mimicking grazing of the components and leguminous of two grass associations with, grazed at two stocking rates.In the cows fistulated to the esophagus, the bite rate was much lower, and the bite size much larger than in the intact animals. The large differences could be due to the different ways of generating such information, since the 8 intact cows were not fed and therefore, their grazing patterns were the usual ones.On the other hand, the two esophageal fistulated cows were fed for several hours prior to sampling, which disrupted their normal grazing behavior patterns. Hess et al (22) compared the legume contents of esophageal fistulated and intact steers when grazing a B.humidicola/rachis. pintoi association and found that fistulated animals selected in favor of legume in the rainy and dry seasons, whereas intact animals selected against legume in the rains, but in favor in the drought. Fistulated steers fed at night before collecting the extrusia, whereas intact steers did not, suggesting the possibility that the nocturnal diet altered steer selectivity.In the present study, cows selected in favor of the legume, which is in agreement with the findings of Ibrahim (21) whose steers behaved similarly. Differences between treatments in CP and DISMO were very evident and can be attributed to the significant contribution of Arachis pintoi to the botanical composition of the extrudate (Table 2, Figure 1). The relationship observed between the Arachis. pintoi content and the CP content of the extrudate is similar to that found by Ibrahim (21), who collected extrudate from esophageal fistulated steers grazing a B. brizantha/A. pintoi association in Costa Rica. This suggests that this legume has the ability to maintain its N content in different ecosystems and management conditions, which is a desirable characteristic if it is desired to improve native grass pastures or degraded pastures of introduced grasses. There are few literature reports on DM or OM intake levels of associated pastures.

In the same experimental station, Fernandez et al (23), used the agronomic method of the difference to estimate dry matter (DM) intake and found no statistical differences between pastures of native grama alone, with a range from 2.53 ± 0.65 to 4.51 ±0.69 kg DM/100 kg DW, and those associated with Arachis. pintoi, whose range was from 2.52 ± 1.05 to 3.34± 0.82 kg DM/100 kg DW. Alonso-Díaz et al (24) used the same technique in a native grass pasture, for a period of three years, and found an average intake of 2.3 ± 1.5 kg DM/100 kg DM/100 kg BW.

In the present study, forage intake of both treatments was within the expected for tropical pastures (25). Arachis pintoi was not able to stimulate forage intake, substituting only the grass. The higher crude protein CP content and higher digestibility of the diet suggested by the analyses carried out on the extrudate of the association would have suggested higher intake, which did not occur.

The net transfer of protein from the feed to the intestines of the grazing ruminant is often not complete and there are ruminal losses when exceeding the value of 210 g of CP/kg of digestible OM (26). In the present study, native pasture (NP) and native pasture plus Arachis pintoi (ANP) presented

165 and 223 g crude protein (CP)/kg digestible organic matter (OM), respectively, suggesting that net losses in crude protein (CP) transfer occurred in the association, due to energy deficiency in the rumen.

It has been stated (26) that if legumes can increase intake by 30%, they could provide enough protein to the intestine to increase milk production by 2.6 kg/cow/day. This did not occur in the present experiment, where intake was lower in the associated pastures.

The inability of Arachis pintoi to improve organic matter (OM) intake suggests that nutritional alternatives should be tested to efficiently use the extra protein consumed by cows.

Adding corn grain to the diet would not only directly increase organic matter (OM) intake, but also provide more digestible energy to avoid wasting crude protein (CP) in the rumen (26). Such The alternative would work at the individual level, but must be economically evaluated before it can be tested experimentally.

The estimation of OM intake from feeding behavior produced lower intake values than the in situ Cr-digestibility technique, being the intake in NP significantly higher than in NAP by 31 % (Table 2). Nevertheless, the intake values by this method are within the wide range expected for tropical pastures (3). The combined use of intact and fistulated cows to estimate grazing time and size of grazing, respectively, caused biases in the intake estimation. Hence, estimates of voluntary intake using intact animals (without surgeries) and markers are the best alternative to study forage intake during grazing.In the associated pasture, cows found more dry matter (DM) present, which allowed them to obtain a larger mouthful than in the control pasture of native grama, reducing their mouthful rate in the first case, and increasing it in the second (Table 2), which led to the feeding rate of native pasture (PN) (24.1 g MO/min) was slightly higher than that of native pasture plus Arachis pintoi (PNA) (21.1 g MO/min); this, in combination with a grazing time only 13 min longer, led to a difference in intake of 1.4 kg MO/cow in favor of the control. Ruminants fed for several hours have a greater drive to graze, evidenced by a higher intake rate, than those animals that have not been fed (27).

Dieting also alters alternate grazing and browsing patterns and leads to longer grazing times, but not to differences in bite size (28). However, Chacon and Stobbs (29) stated that the effect of nocturnal dieting was small compared to pasture characteristics, but indicated that the dieting time should be the minimum necessary to obtain a satisfactory feeding rate. In addition, the sampling protocol should interrupt grazing only for the time necessary to place collection bags and obtain esophageal extrusion. Brazilian researchers have good results have been obtained by not feeding fistulated cows to the esophagus (30, 31).The shorter rumination time presented by the association would have suggested a faster physical degradation of the grazed forage and consequently a higher intake, as a result of a faster rate of passage of the feed, which did not occur. Therefore, in associated pastures of grasses and herbaceous legumes such as the present one, it is necessary to study which factors affect the speed with which ingested forage passes through the animal's gastrointestinal tract and which are limiting consumption.

The time the experimental animals were off pasture averaged 265 min/day; transit to and from the milking parlor was 30 min, about 10 min at milking and 60 min to nurse the calf. This left a lot of "dead" time both before cows were milked and after nursing; this period is much longer than the milking period of 120 to 130 min reported by Cowan (32).This factor undoubtedly reduced the grazing time of the cows in the present study. A grazing experiment of short duration such as the present one is not representative of the animal productive performance of a complete production cycle (33). However, it allows relating short-term performance to pasture characteristics that allow identifying the type of management options that optimize forage acquisition by the ruminant (25). Differences between treatments in saleable milk and milk consumed by the calf were not significant, but were significant in total milk.

The higher nutrient intake of the associated pasture due to a higher nutritive value was the factor responsible for this difference (34). The nutritive value of the esophageal extrusa of the cows that grazed the association was superior to that of the native grasses without legume.However, there were no differences between treatments in organic matter (OM) intake, so crude protein (CP) and digestible organic matter (DOM) intake was higher in the association, and consequently, total milk production was higher. This type of study should consider climatic variability within and between years. For this reason, it should be carried out in representative climatic periods (rains, northeast, drought) and repeated for at least two years. This will allow us to corroborate if introducing the legume to the native pasture is a viable alternative to increase milk and calf production in dual-purpose systems in the Mexican tropics.

TABLES AND FIGURES

Relationship between *Arachis Pintoi* content with crude protein and in situ dry matter digestibility.

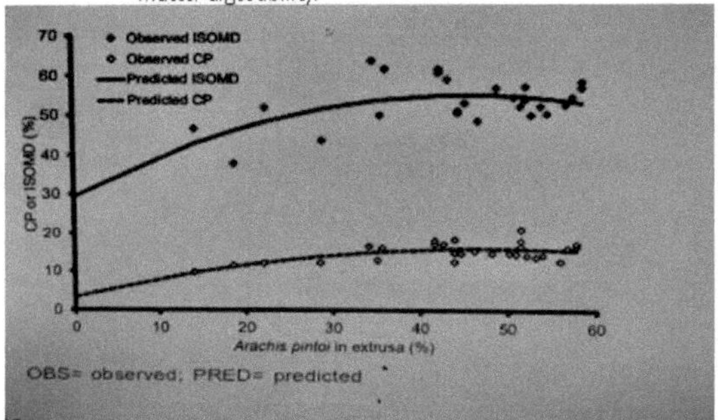

Individual milk production measurements in native grass pastures or pastures associated with *Arachis Pintoi*.

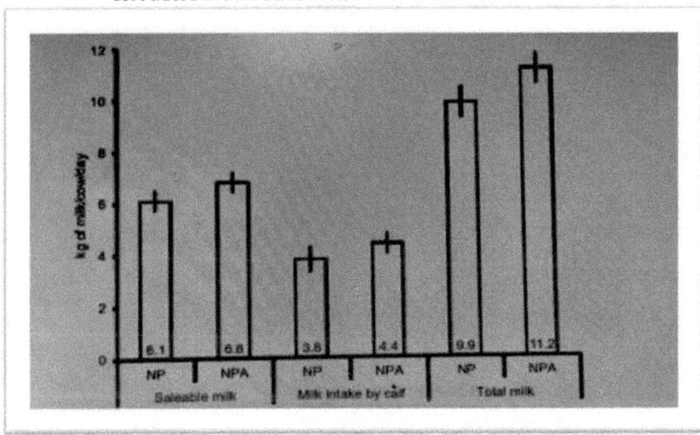

The lines above the bars are the standard errors.

PICTURES

Table 1. Historical averages of precipitation and minimum and maximum temperatures, as well as those occurring during the experiment.

Experiment al period	History (1980-1999)			Experimental (2000)		
	PP. in mm.	Tem. Min.o C	Tem. M áx oC	PP. in mm.	Tem. Min.o C	Tem. M áx oC
Period 1 (25 Jun to July 15		22.6	31.6		21.4	33.4
Period2.25 Jul to 14 Aug		22.5	31.3	142	20.9	33.3

Dry matter present before grazing and botanical composition of native grass pastures alone or associated with Arachis pintoi. ab Means with the same letter in a row are statistically different (P<0.05).

Variables	Native grasses	Native grasses/Arachis pintoi
Average dry matter present before grazing (Kg/ha)	3314 ± 212a	4225 ± 212b
Botanical composition % Arachis pintoi CIAT 17434	----------------------	28.3 ± 3.9b
Native grasses	58.7 ± 2.1a	45.0 ± 2.1b
Introduced grasses	10.2 ± 1.5a	4.3 ± 1.5b
Savannah grass Sporobolus poiretii	11.7 ± 1.2a	5.2 ± 1.2b
Paspalum bittergrass virgatum	2.8 ± 0.7a	4.1 ± 0.7a
Broadleaf weeds	10.1 ± 0.7a	6.9 ± 0.7 b
Native legume	6.6 ± 0.9 a	6.2 ± 0.9a

Table 3. Treatment means for ingestive behavior, esophageal extrusion and consumption variables.

Variable	Native grasses	Native grasses/ Arachis pintoi
Esophageal extrusion		
Arachis pintoi, %, %.	0.0 ± 0.0 a	43.6 ± 2.3 b
Pastures % Pasture	98.2 ± 2.4 a	56.0 ± 1.8 b
Native grasses % native grasses % native grasses % native grasses	% 1.7 ± 0.2 a	0.0 ± 0.0 b
Other species % Other species	0.1 ± 0.5 a	0.4 ± 0.1 a
Crude protein % of DM.	10.6 ± 0.5 a	15.1 ± 0.4 b
In situ digestibility of MO %.	64.1 ± 2.4 a	67.6 ± 1.7 b
Ingestion Behavior		
Grazing time in min/day	380 ± 11.0 a	367 ± 11.0 a
Ruminating time min/day	379 ± 8.0 a	291 ± 8.0 b
Time in other activities minutes /day	677 ± 14.0 a	776 ±14.0 b
Bite speed, bites/min	35.4 ± 1.0 a	22.0 ± 1.1 b
Bite size, g /bite MO	0.68 ± 0.06 a	0.96 ± 0.04 b
Dry matter consumption		
In situ digestibility C2 (kg MO/100 kg PV)	0.68 ± 0.06 a	2.09 ± 0.11 a
Behavior of feed (kg MO/100 kg PV)	2.02 ± 0.12 a	1.54 ± 0.12 b

Ab Means with the same letter in a row are statistically different (P<0.05).

LITERATURE CITED

1. Wade MH, Carvalho PCF. Defoliation patterns and herbage intake on pastures. In: Lemaire G, et al, editors. Grassland ecophysiology and grazing ecology. 1st ed. 1st ed. Wallingsford,UK: CABI Publishing; 2000:233-248.

2. Penning PD, Rutter SM. Ingestive behavior. In: Leaver JD, editor. Herbage intake handbook. 2nd ed. Hurley, UK: The British Grassland Society;2004: 151-175.

3. Minson DJ. Forage in Ruminant Nutrition. 1st edition. New York, USA: Academic Press; 1990.

4. Carulla JE, Lascano CE, Ward, JK. Selectivity of residentand oesophageal fistulated steers grazing Arachis pintoiand Brachiaria dictyoneura in the Llanos of Colombia. Trop Grasslds 1991; 25:317-324.

5. Hernández M, Argel PJ, Ibrahim MA, Mannetje L. 't. Pasture production, diet selection and liveweight gains of cattle grazing Brachiaria brizantha with or without Arachis pintoi at two stocking rates in the Atlantic Zone of Costa Rica.Trop Grasslds 1995; 29: 134-141.

6. Hess HD, Kreuzer M, Nösberger J, Wenk C, Lascano CE. (2002). Effect of sward attributes on legume selection by oesophageal-fistulated and non- fistulated steers grazing tropical grass-legume pasture. Trop Grasslds 2002; 36:227-238.

7. Castillo GE, Braulio Valles MB, Mannetje L 't, Aluja SA. Effect of introducing Arachis pintoi on soil variables of native grass pastures of the Mexican humid tropics Téc Pecu Méx 2005;43: 287-295. Ørskov ER, McDonald I. The estimation of protein degradability in the rumen from incubation measurements eighted according to rate of passage. J Agric Sci Camb1979; 92:499-503.

16. Statistical Analysis System. SAS/STAT® Software: Changes and Enhancements. Release 8.1. Cary, NC: SAS Institute Inc.; 2000.

17. Mott GO. Grazing pressure and the measurement of pasture production. Proc VIII International Grassland Congress. 1960:606-611.

18. Mannetje L 't. Relations between pasture attributes and liveweight gains on a sub-tropical pasture. In: Iglovikov VG, Movsissiants AP, editors. Proc XII International Grassland Congress. Moscow, Soviet Union. 1974, Vol. III: 299- 304.

19. Monsalve LRA, Sosa MC, Castillo GE, Jarillo RJ, Aluja SA, Mannetje L 't. Effect of associating native grasses with Arachis pintoi CIAT 17434 on ingestive behavior of dual-purpose cows [abstract]. National Livestock Research Meeting. 2000:89.

20. Cowan RT, O'Grady P. Effect of presentation yield of a tropical grass-legume pasture on grazing time and milk yield of Friesian cows. Trop Grasslds 1976;10:213-218.

21. Ibrahim MA. Compatibility, persistence and productivity of grass-legume mixtures for sustainable animal production in the Atlantic Zone of Costa Rica. [doctoral thesis] Wageningen, The Netherlands: Wageningen Agricultural University; 1994.

22. Hess HD, Kreuzer M, Nösberger J, Wenk C, Lascano CE.

Effect of sward attributes on legume selection by oesophageal-fistulated and non-fistulated steers grazing tropical grass-legume pasture. Trop Grasslds 2002; 36:227-238.
23. Fernández TL, Castillo GE, Ocaña ZE, Valles MB, Jarillo RJ. Vegetation characteristics in native grasses alone or associated with
Arachis pintoi CIAT 17434 in intensive rotational grazing. Téc Pecu Méx 2006;44:365-378.
24. Alonso DMA, Castillo GE, Basurto CH, Jarillo RJ, Valles MB. Productive response of a native grass pasture.

CHAPTER III

Effect of introducing Arachis pintoi on soil variables of native grass pastures in the Mexican humid tropics.

Epigmenio Castillo Gallegosa,, Braulio Valles de la Mora†, Leendert 't Mannetje and Eliazar Ocaña Zavaleta.

INTRODUCTION

The native grasses were formed by clearing and burning the original forest, followed by several cycles of crops such as corn, which relatively quickly depleted the soil's natural nutrient reserves. When the volume of crops was reduced, the option for producers was to graze the land by domestic cattle, whose effect, together with periodic burning, resulted in a savanna vegetation, dominated by grasses of the genera Setaria and Cynodon, complemented by leguminous plants of the genera Macroptylium, Desmodium and Centrosema (1).This vegetation covers between 25 and 75 % of the pastures in Mexico's humid tropics, and is the main source of feed for cattle and dual-purpose cattle. In practice, these lands are not fertilized nor do they have productive legumes that add adequate amounts of nitrogen, which is the driving element of pasture growth, which, after dozens of years of use, has led to the degradation of soil and pasture fertility. In the future, the viability of the native grass agroecosystem will depend on its capacity to provide environmental services, such as effective carbon sequestration, which would contribute to the reduction of atmospheric CO2 (2).The establishment and maintenance of introduced grasses is expensive because the cost of the seed is high, in addition to the fact that their permanence in the pasture and their productive level depend to a great extent on the availability of nitrogen. For this reason, it is quite probable that introduced grasses are adopted on a low scale by cattle farmers in the tropical region, because they do not fertilize or associate persistent and compatible legumes with introduced grasses. Therefore, we propose that the sustainable improvement of native grass pastures in the humid tropics of Mexico can be achieved through the use of persistent legumes that improve soil fertility through biological N2 fixation, and simultaneously increase animal production by improving the nutritional quality of the diet of domestic ruminants.Arachis pintoi CIAT 17434 is a legume that has increased milk and meat production through its association with introduced grasses such as African star grass (Cynodon plectostachyus, and Santo Domingo star grass C. nlemfuensis) and Brachiaria spp (3,4), as well as improving soil N and C inventories (5). The present work describes the effect of the introduction of the perennial forage legume Arachis pintoi CIAT 17434 in native grasses on some soil variables considered important for the sustainability of the pasture agroecosystem.

MATERIAL AND METHODS

The study was conducted at the Centro de Enseñanza, Investigación y Extensión en Ganadería Tropical (CEIEGT) of the Facultad de Medicina Veterinaria y Zootecnia of the Universidad Nacional Autónoma de México, located in the coastal plain of the Gulf of Mexico, 40 km west of the coastline, at 20° 02' N, 97° 06' W, and 112 masl. The climate (1980-2000) is warm and humid with year-round rainfall, with average annual precipitation of 1931 ± 334 mm. Average monthly rainfall is highly variable (161 ± 132 mm), but generally sufficient for pasture growth, as droughts tend to be occasional and short. The average daily mean temperature was 23.9 ± 6.4 °C.Average monthly maximum (29.2 ± 3.3 °C) and minimum (18.6 ± 3.9 °C) temperatures are reasonably uniform from year to year. The climatic seasons are: rainy, from July to October, with precipitation and high temperature; winter or "nortes" from November to February, with rain and decreasing temperatures, and "drought", from March to June. Low temperatures in winter and high evapotranspiration in drought do not favor forage production, particularly the latter, since the shallow soil of the experimental site does not store much moisture. The soils are Ultisols (Durustults) clay-loam, acidic, and with low concentrations of P (3.5 ppm by Bray and 2.0 ppm by Olsen), S, Ca and K, as well as low cation exchange capacity (10.5 meq/100 g), aluminum saturation does not reach toxic levels for plants (6,7). There is an impermeable layer between 0 and 25 cm deep, which causes inadequate drainage during rain and winter.In 1998, samples from the experimental area indicated that carbon (C) decreased from 1.02 ± 0.44 % at 0 to 15 cm to 0.78 ± 0.15 % at 15 to 30 cm, as did nitrogen (N), with 0.13 ± 0.06 and 0.10 ± 0.04 %. Two treatments were established: native grasses (NG) and NG + Arachis pintoi in which Arachis pintoi CIAT 17434 (NG+Ap) was vegetatively sown at 1.0 m between furrows and 0.5 m between plants.The first field (C1) of the association was established between August and November 2006, which was grazed lightly and intermittently between May and August 2007 and has been grazed without interruption since then. Field 2 (C2) was established in November 1998, and was only excluded from grazing for 30 days following legume planting. In both cases, the stolons were planted without soil preparation and only in C1 was glyphosate applied to reduce competition to the newly planted legume.Each field had seven permanent divisions of 22 m wide by 165 m long, which in turn were temporarily subdivided into three sections of 22 m by 55 m (21 sections in total), to carry out rotational grazing of one day of grazing and 20 days of recovery. The stocking rate (CA) was 2 cows/ha during the period of low forage production and 3.2 cows/ha the rest of the year. Stocking rate (LR) was reduced when dry matter present before grazing decreased to less than 2,500 kg/ha in any section sampled. Seven transepts, one per division, were established in April 2009 and September 2010, placed at the center of the division and along the entire length of the division, and six soil samples were collected at equal distances in each transept. A total of 336 soil samples were obtained and analyzed for the variables described below. To estimate bulk density (DA, g/cm3), a metal cylinder (50 mm internal diameter and 50 mm height) was introduced into the bare soil; the cylinder was recovered with soil and dried at 65° C until constant weight (8). The remaining samples were dried at room temperature, roots and other organic material were removed and ground to pass a 2 mm sieve. The pH was measured with a potentiometer, in soil (two parts) suspended in distilled water (one part). Organic carbon (C, %) was analyzed according to the Walkley and Black technique (9).Organic matter (OM, %) was calculated assuming a 58 % C content in OM (8). Total C (Ct, kg/ha) for the 0 to 20 cm layer was calculated with the equation: Ct = Vs x DA x C/100, where: Vs is the volume in 1 ha at 20 cm depth, DA is the bulk density (kg/m3), and C was already defined. The DA of the 0 to 5 cm layer was assumed to be representative of that of the 0 to 20 cm layer. Nitrogen (N, %) was estimated with the Kjeldahl technique, calculating total nitrogen (Nt, kg/ha) in a similar way to total carbon (CT)t, substituting C for N.Every three months, the contribution of Arachis. pintoi to the botanical composition was evaluated in field 1 in two sections of each of the three divisions selected for sampling, as they were visually the most representative of the field. Sections b1, d1 and f1 had a higher content of Arachis. pintoi, compared to the other three (b3, d3 and f3), being named as high and low in legume, respectively. The division was considered as the experimental unit, so the variation between sampling points within the transect was omitted. The analysis of variance was performed separately for C1 and C2. The additive linear model used was the following:

$Yijk = M + Tj + Di (Tj) + Ak + (T \times A)jk + Eijk$, where:

Yijk is the response variable, recorded in the transect corresponding to the i-th division, within the j-th treatment, in the k-th year; M is the overall mean common to all observations; Tj is the effect of the jth treatment (j: GN and GN+Ap); Di (Tj) is the variation between divisions within the jth treatment, used as an error to test the treatment effect; Ak is the effect of the kth year (k: 1999 and 2000); (T x A) jk is the combined effect, or interaction, of treatment by year; and, Eijk is the residual variation, used as an error to test the year and interaction effects. Because the samples were taken at different times each year, it was decided to omit the annual means from the presentation of results, in order to concentrate on the treatment means.

RESULTS

The T x A interaction did not affect (P>0.05) any response variable, so the main effects of T and A were independent.In C1, the effect of T was not significant on pH and DA, and was only 6 thousandths away from being significant on C:N (P=0.0563), and was significant (P<0.05) on the other variables; while in C2, T did not affect any variable (Table 1), which is explained by the fact of the different establishment time of each field, which indicated that the legume needs a medium term to start showing its beneficial effects on the soil. The contribution of Arachis. pintoi to the botanical composition increased linearly in the sections with high and low initial legume content. The increase in the former was 13.3 percentage units per year; and in the latter, the value was 7.8 (Figure 1).Increase in the contribution of Arachis pintoi to botanical composition in field 1, in three sections with low initial content and three sections with high initial content.

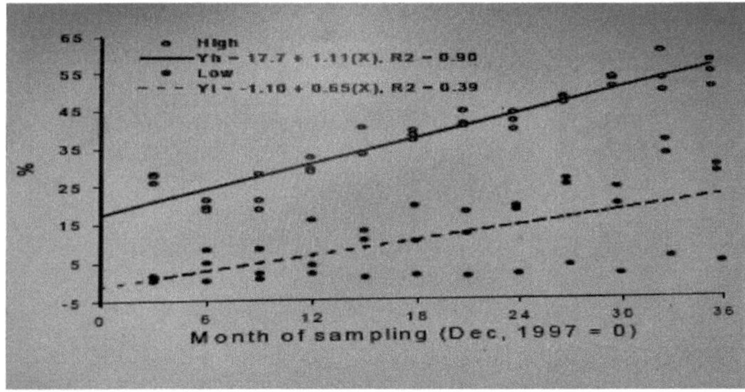

The respective contribution of the legume, when sampling the soil, indicated a slight relationship with the respective carbon and nitrogen contents; although the high variation did not allow finding significant associations (Table 2). An important aspect of productivity in tropical pastures is to maintain or increase the soil C and N inventory, in response to increases in biomass, induced by biological N fixation[2] , which implies long-term sequestration of CO2, as well as an increase in soil fertility. However, there are also negative effects of biological nitrogen fixation, such as soil acidification, which only manifest themselves in the long term (10). Legumes reduce soil compaction, which results from increasing animal stocking rates (11), but in the present study, three and a half years after establishment, there was no effect of Arachis. pintoi on soil compaction. In Costa Rica, Ibrahim (5) found that by increasing animal stocking rate from 2 to 3 AU/ha in a Brachiaria spp/A. pintoi association, DA increased only slightly from 0.76 to 0.85 g/cm3 in the 0 to 5 cm soil layer. It has been found (12,13) that A. pintoi CIAT 17434 derived 65 to 85 % of its N from fixation, indicating N accumulation in the soil, which increases the probability of NO3 leaching and soil acidification (10). However, in the present experiment, the presence of Arachis. pintoi in the soil was not long enough to influence pH.Valles (13) sampled the soil profile in both treatments up to 1 m depth in C1, when Arachis pintoi was one year old, and did not detect differences in the pH of the profiles. However, in native grasses associated for five years with the legume, pH was significantly (P<0.05) lower at all depths than that of grasses without legume. The respective pH values for the former, at depths of 0-5, 5-15 and 15-30 cm, were 5.05, 5.07 and 5.52; and in the latter they were 5.66, 5.44 and 5.72. This suggests that there is a risk of a future decrease in soil pH in the Arachis pintoi/native gram association.

Table 1. Effect of pasture on soil variables at the two sowing sites (mean ± standard error).

Variable	Pasture Native grass alone	Pasture Native grass +. Arachis p.
Field 1		
Ph	Ph 5.12±0.05 a	5.17±0.04 a
Bulk density g/cm3 1	22±0.02 a	1.24±0.02 a
Organic matter %a	2.27±0.10a	2.53±0.09 b
Organic carbon, %, organic carbon, %, organic carbon, %, organic carbon, %, organic carbon, %, organic carbon	1.32±0.06 a	1.47±0.05 b
Nitrogen, % x 10-2 a	14.15±1.39a	22.43±2.02 b
Sampling of Carbon and:Nitrogen in units)	12.40±1.38 a	.46.00±1.11 a
Carbon in soil, kg/ha	31968±1285 a	36197±1144 b
Nitrogen in soil, kg/ha	3452±341 a	5610±526 b
Field 2		
pH	5.03±0.04 a	5.12±0.05 a
Bulk density, g/cm3	1.17±0.03 a	1.21±0.02 a
Organic matter, %, organic matter, %, %, organic matter, %, organic matter, %, organic matter, %, organic matter	2.61±0.12 a	2.67±0.15 a
Organic carbon, % a	1.52±0.07a	1.55±0.09 a
nitrogen, % x 10-2	10.45±1.35 a	11.99±1.27 a
C:N ratio (without units)	22.19±2.41a	18.96±1.83 a
Coal in soil (Total carbon, kg/ha)	35783±2179 a	37847±2493 a
nitrogen in soil (N), kg/ha)	2420±298 a	2861±285 a

Ab Means with deferent super index statistically different (P<0.05).

Table 2. Contribution of Arachis pintoi to botanical composition, and amounts (kg/ha) of organic carbon and nitrogen contained in the soil at a depth of 0.2 m (mean ± standard error; n = 6).

Initial percentage of Arachis pintoi	Sampling of soil in A. pintoi at (%)	Soil carbon sampling kg/ha	Soil nitrogen sampling (kg/ha)
Under	17 ± 6.0 a	32,524 ± 10,871 a	4,929 ± 2,416 a
High	46 ± 4.5 b	43,420 ± 5,424 a	5,667 ± 2,474 a

Ab Means with different super index are different (P<0.05).

The continuous addition of roots and leaf litter, together with a chronic N deficiency, are the factors responsible for the accumulation of OM in the soil of the pasture agroecosystem (14). An initial (1998) Ct value was calculated for both treatments of 24.7 t/ha; and by linear regression, an average annual increase until year 2,000, of 3.7 and 4.8 t/ha/year for GN and GN+Ap, respectively, which was an acceptable differential increase. This is in agreement with the observations of Fisher et al.(15) in the Colombian savanna, and of Ibrahim in the Costa Rican humid tropics (5).The carbon (c) to nitrogen (N) ratio is an indicator of soil quality, with a value of 10:1 or less being considered ideal. In C1, native grasses (NG) exceeded the ideal value, but that of the association was slightly lower (Table 1). In contrast, in carbon (C2), both treatments showed values well above the ideal.This difference must be due to the different time of legume establishment in both fields. In Costa Rica (5), the soil C:N ratio of a Brachiaria spp/A. pintoi association was found to be 12.5:1, comparable to those of the C1 control treatment of the present study, but lower than the data reported for C2. This suggests that the legume, in addition to remaining productive in the association, needs sufficient time to improve the soil C:N ratio. It was concluded that three and a half years after its introduction into native grass pastures, Arachis pintoi CIAT 17434 induced increases in soil carbon and nitrogen contents, which is indicative of its ability to improve fertility and thereby maintain the sustainability of tropical dual-purpose livestock systems.

LITERATURE CITED

1. Bosman HG, Castillo GE, Valles MB, De Lucía GR. Botanical composition and nodulation of legumes in native pastures of the Gulf of Mexico coastal plain. Pasturas Tropicales 1990;12(1):2-8.

2. Westerhof R, Vilela L, Ayarza MA, Zech W. Carbon Fractions as Sensitive Indicators of Quality of Soil Organic Matter. In: Thomas R, Ayarza MA editors. Sustainable land management for the oxisols of the Latin American Savannas - Dynamics of soil organic matter and indicators of soil quality. Cali, Colombia: International Center for Tropical Agriculture; CIAT Publication. No. 312; 1999:131-140.

3. González MS, Van Heurck LM, Romero F, Pezo DA, Argel PJ. Milk production in African star (Cynodon nlemfuensis) pastures alone and associated with Arachis pintoi or Desmodium ovalifolium. Pasturas Tropicales 1996; 18(1):2-12.

4. Hernández M, Argel PJ, Ibrahim MA, 't Mannetje L. Pasture production, diet selection and liveweight gains of cattle grazing Brachiaria brizantha with or without Arachis pintoi at two stocking rates in the Atlantic Zone of Costa Rica. Tropical Grasslands 1995; 29(3):134-141.

5. Ibrahim MA. Compatibility, persistence and productivity of grass-legume mixtures for sustainable animal production in the Atlantic Zone of Costa Rica [PhD Thesis]. Wageningen, The Netherlands; Wageningen Agricultural University; 1994.

6. Arscott TG. Soils of the CIEEGT. Soil Consultancy Report to the Project: Research, Teaching and Extension in Tropical Livestock, FAO, Rome, Italy/CIEEGT, FMVZ, UNAM, Martinez de la Torre, Veracruz, Mexico [Internal circulation]. 1978.

7. Toledo JM. Tropical Legume Research Plan for CIEEGT, Martinez de la Torre, Veracruz, Mexico. Tropical Pasture Consultancy Report for the Project: Teaching and Extension for Milk and Meat Production in the Tropics. FAO, Rome, Italy /CIEEGT, FMVZ, UNAM, Martínez de la Torre, Veracruz, Mexico [Internal circulation]. 1986.

8. Anderson JM, Ingram JSI. Tropical soil biology and fertility: Handbook of methods, 2nd ed. Wallingford, UK: CAB International; 1993.

9. Walkley A, Black TA. An examination of the Degtjareff method for determining soil organic matter and a proposed modification of the chromic acid titration method. Soil Sci 1934; 37(1):29-38.

10. Haynes RJ. Soil acidification induced by leguminous crops. Grass Forage Sci 1983; 38(1):1-11.

11. Alegre JC, Lara PD. Effect of grazing animals on the physical properties of soils in the humid tropical region of Peru. Pasturas Tropicales 1991;13(1):18-23.

12. Thomas RJ, Asakawa NM, Rondon MA, Alarcon HF. Nitrogen fixation by three tropical forage legumes in acid-soil savanna of Colombia. Soil Biol Biochem 1997; 29(5-6):801-808.

13. Valles MB. Contribution of the forage legume Arachis pintoi to soil fertility in a tropical pasture system in Veracruz, Mexico [PhD Thesis]. London, UK: University of London; 2001.

14. Huntjes JLM, Albers RAJM. A model experiment to study the influence of living plants on the accumulation of soil organic matter in pastures. Plant Soil 1978; (50):411-418.

15. Fisher MJ, Rao IM, Ayarza MA, Lascano CE Sanz JI, Thomas RJ, Vera RR. Carbon storage by introduced deep-rooted grasses in the South American savannas. Nature 1994; (371): 236-238.

CHAPTER IV

Nitrogen mineralization in Arachis pinto pasture soils

Braulio Valles de la Mora†, Georg Cadisch, Epigmenio Castillo Gallegos

INTRODUCTION

In the humid tropics of Mexico, native pastures (Paspalum spp, Axonopus spp, Cynodon spp, mainly) are the basis of the animal production system known as "dual purpose", in which producers manage different types of cattle, in extensive and continuous grazing, having meat and milk as their main products.(1) Pasture productivity depends on mineralized N, as well as other important nutrients (P, Ca and K); and efficient residue decomposition and N release, which in turn depends on the C:N ratio associated with nutrient requirements for decomposing organisms. Nitrogen (N) availability in legume-based pastures as well as in crop/pasture rotation is higher than in native savannas and continuous cropping systems (2). Other authors showed that high potential nitrogen (N) mineralization rates (anaerobic incubation, 40 °C, 7 d) have been achieved in an Oxisol soil (clayey, organic matter 3.4 % and total N of 1008 ppm), under greenhouse conditions, in a Brachiaria decumbens + Pueraria phaseoloides pasture (6.84 g N g-1 soil d-1) compared to Brachiaria decumbens pasture alone (3.86 g N g-1 soil d-1), and that the legume contributed 29 % of the total soil carbon found in the first 2 cm depth (3). Nitrogen (N) mineralization is strongly dependent on the ability of the legume to fix N2, and the importance of this biological process is to improve the supply of available soil nitrogen (N).The ability of legumes to fix atmospheric nitrogen (N) is due to a symbiotic relationship with bacteria of the genus Rhizobium. In this relationship, both the plant and the bacteria contribute and receive benefits as a result of their association. Bacteria that perform the role of atmospheric N fixation are host specific, and many tropical legumes are highly specific in their associations with rhizobia (4). Also, the amount of N2 fixed is affected by the efficiency of Rhizobium spp strains in establishing a functional association with the host. Some symbioses may not be effective even if there is abundant nodulation (5), but the development of inoculants has allowed the successful introduction of legumes to new agricultural systems where compatible rhizobia were absent from the soil (6). The genus Arachis has been classified as effectively promiscuous, meaning that its species will nodulate effectively with a wide range of Rhizobium. Arachis pintoi Krapov. & Greg. has shown high efficiency when nodulated with Bradyrhizobium strain CIAT 3101(7) as well as with native strains(8). Little information is available on nitrogen (N) mineralization in soils with forage legumes associated with native pastures. in the Mexican humid tropics.Arachis pintoi is a species whose leaf litter decomposes rapidly in the soil

(9,10). It was introduced to the north-central region of the state of Veracruz, Mexico in 1986 (11), and in evaluations carried out during two years with other legumes, it was one of the most promising species for this ecosystem (12,13). Therefore, the objective of this study was to compare the N mineralization of an Ultisol soil with native pastures associated with A. pintoi CIAT 17434 against native pastures alone, using aerobic and anaerobic laboratory techniques.

MATERIAL AND METHODS

Four sites of the Centro de Enseñanza, Investigación y Extensión en Ganadería Tropical (CEIEGT) belonging to the Facultad de Medicina Veterinaria y Zootecnia (Universidad Nacional Autónoma de México) were used. CEIEGT is located in the coastal plain of the Gulf of Mexico, 40 km from the coast, at 20° 02' N and 97° 06' W, at 112 m asl. At these sites, Arachis pintoi IATTC 17434 was established from 3, 5, 8, and 11 years ago. The sites were identified as S3(4.0 ha), S5 (10.0 ha), S8 (0.5 ha) and S11 (0.25 ha), together with pastures without legumes, selected as controls. In both groups of sites, soils were sampled in June-August 1997. Prior to laboratory analysis, the samples were kept in black plastic bags and stored in a dry environment to avoid any effect on the mineralization results. Some of the characteristics of these soils are presented in Table 1. In S3 and S5 the legume was introduced to form associations with grasses: the former was associated within a native pasture (3 years-Arachis. pintoi), and the latter, with African star - Cynodon nlemfuensis- (5 years-Arachis. pintoi) at the same time. At sites S8 and S11, Arachis. pintoi was planted in monoculture as seed banks.The legume was not inoculated, but in the four sites, a profuse inoculation of rhizobia of native strains was observed. The control areas corresponded to soils with native vegetation dominated by grasses of the genera Paspalum, Axonopus and Cynodon; and by legumes (<10 % of the area) mainly of the genera Desmodium and Calopogonium, which were under rotational grazing at the time of sampling, except control S8, which remained unused. The S11 control remained in grazing until two years prior to sampling. Soils were unfertilized Ultisols for at least five years prior to and during the experiment.The site for each treatment was divided into four plots and a soil subsample was obtained from each plot using a auger. The four sub-samples for each depth were mixed to form a composite sample.Sampling depths were 0-5, 5-15 and 15-30 cm for anaerobic incubation (ANA), and 0-5 and 5-15 cm for aerobic incubation (AER). To determine the N released by the anaerobic incubation method (ANA), a modification of the technique of Waring and Bremner (14) was used. Ten g of dry soil were weighed, placed in test tubes, to which 15 ml of distilled water was added. The tubes were sealed and kept at 40 °C for seven days. (time 7). At the end of the incubation, ammonium was extracted by adding 30 ml of 3M KCl to the soils. The samples were shaken and filtered prior to NH4 + analysis by colorimetry with an autoanalyzer. The same procedure was performed before incubation to determine mineral nitrogen (N) at zero time. To calculate the nitrogen (N) released, the following formula(15) was used: Potential nootrogen mineralization rate N= (µg NH4 +-N g-1 soil, time 7 days) - (µg NH4 + -N g-1 soil, time 0 days)/7 days To develop the aerobic incubation method (AER), soil samples (60 g) of 0-5 and 5-15 cm depth, from sites S3, S5 and S8, and their corresponding control treatments, were used, placed in columns (3 cm diameter tubes, 25 cm long) at 28 °C. At baseline, and subsequently at 7, 21, 49, 114, 231, and 301 days of incubation, the soils were percolated with 150 ml (in 50-ml increments) of a solution containing 1 mm MgSO4, 1 mm CaCl2, 0.9 mm KCl, and

0.1 mm KH2PO4 (16).Ammonium and nitrate were analyzed by colorimetry with an autoanalyzer, according to the following equation (15): mineralized N= (µg NO3+NH4 sample - µg NO3+NH4 blank)/g soil Data from both experiments were analyzed separately, as a split-plot design using soils (with or without the legume) as the major plot and depths as subplots, repeated four (ANA) or three (AER) times. Analyses of variance were performed using mineralization rates and accumulated mineralized N as response variables. Comparisons of means were made using DMS. To describe mineralization trends, the data were fitted (17) to simple exponential curves approximating the maximum value. To choose the equation that best described the trends, the R2 value was used as a criterion, and the equation chosen was: Y = y0 + a(1-e-bx) Where Y is the N mineralized at time x; y0 is the N mineralized when x = 0; a is the asymptote or maximum N mineralized, reached as x → ∞; and b is the rate of nitrogen (N) mineralization.

Anaerobic incubation

The ANA results were atypical and inconsistent. The highest mineralization rate was expected in soils planted with the introduced legume, rather than with the native pasture, where at these sites the native legume population has been estimated to be very poor (7.1 %) (18). Mineralization data will always correspond to µg NH4 +-N g-1 soil d-1. Considering the ANA results, in S3 there were differences in anaerobic potential mineralization between pastures with Arachis. pintoi and its control, at the three depths (Table 2). The average of the three depths was 3.1±0.7 (pastures with Arachis pintoi) vs 10.4±1.3 µg (native pastures) (P0.05). At S5 the differences in anaerobic mineralization between native pasture soils (6.2±1.4 µg) and soils with the legume (7.5±1.5 µg) were not significant (Table 2).In all cases the mineralization rate decreased with depth, averaging for both soils (with and without the forage legume) 10.6±1.8, 6.1±1.5 and 3.1± 0.7 µg (P≤0.05) at 0-5, 5-15 and 15-30 cm. Only in S5 at 0-5 cm was there a slightly higher value compared to the native pasture soil (11.6 vs. 10.6 µg), respectively. As in S5, N mineralized from site S8 with A. pintoi was not significantly different from native pasture soils (8.9±2.3 µg) and with Arachis pintoi (6.5±1.9 µg); however, there were significant differences (P≤0.001) between 0-5 cm (14.4±3.1) and the shallowest depths (5.7±0.6 and 3.1±1.0 µg at 5-15 and 15-30 cm). At S11, the control showed a high N mineralization rate (9.0±1.4 µg), different (P<0.001).In the nutrient uptake process, the rhizosphere is very important, particularly in conditions of low fertility; and the fibrous roots of grasses affect nitrogen (N) mineralization (19). In S11 these results were even more unexpected, as the site had close to 100 % legume cover; however, the control produced 2.7 times more mineral N than the soil with the introduced legume. In S5 and S8 the pastures with A. pintoi produced on average 6.3±1.1 µg, which is only 70 % of the N produced by the soil with native pasture alone (9.0±5.7 µg). In the Cerrado brasileño, data. potential N mineralization (incubation at 40 °C, 7 d) in various land use systems, ranging from native pastures (savanna) to continuous cropping systems on Oxisols soils (20) have shown that, contrary to our results, potentially mineralizable nitrogen (N) was highest in associated Brachiaria decumbens/Stylosanthes guianensis pastures (63 kg N ha-1), followed by Brachiaria decumbens alone (43 kg N ha-1), no-till continuous cropping (26 kg N ha-1), native savanna (23 kg N ha-1) and continuous cropping with conventional tillage (18 kg N ha-1). These authors mentioned that the presence of the legume promoted microbial activity, and therefore more N was mineralized. Other authors found that the introduction of Stylosanthes spp. in an Andropogon gayanus pasture had a positive effect on potentially mineralizable nitrogen (N). They estimated that the associated pasture, at a soil depth of 0-5 cm, produced 20.3 µg N g-1 soil, compared with the grass pasture alone (11.6 µg N g-1 soil) (21).In our study, the trend of decreasing nitrogen (N) mineralization with depth was consistent across all sites, although correlation coefficients (R2) between soil depth and mineralization were not high: 0.36 and 0.50 for sites with Arachis. pintoi and native pastures, respectively.

Several studies have shown that the net nitrogen mineralization

(N) decreases with increasing depth, and they have mentioned that above 20 cm it accounts for as much as 75 % (22) or 61 % (23) of the total. However, the relative importance of net mineralization from the subsoil may be high during dry periods when moisture limitations are present in the surface layer, but not in the subsoil (24). Aerobic incubation Mineralization data will always correspond to µg N g-1 soil.Referring to aerobic incubation (AER), in S3 N mineralization values were different (PP<0.001) between native pasture and pasture with Arachis. pintoi, both at 0-5 cm (159±2.4 vs 131±1.4 µg) and at 5-15 cm depth (92±1.0 vs 77± 0.8 µg). At this site, the soils at 5-15 cm mineralized, on average, only 58 % (84±1.2 µg) of the mineralized nitrogen (N) at 0-5 cm (145±2.1 µg; P<0.001; Figure 1).In the pasture with Arachis. pintoi from S5, differences (P<0.001) were found only for depth: 226±4.0 and 148±2.5 µg for 0-5 and 5-15 cm, respectively. Soil with Arachis. pintoi mineralized 207±3.4 µg in 43 weeks, compared to 166±3.1 µg from the site in the native pasture (Figure 2). The cumulative values resulted in 19 and 26 % with more N mineralized from the sites with Arachis. pintoi than from the sites with native pasture at 0-5 cm and 5- 15 cm depth; however, these differences were not significant. In S8, mineralization was found only in the Arachis. pintoi seedbed, as sufficient soil was not available for the control site (Figure 3). The average values of the six percolates were 239±3.2 and 178±3.5 µg at 0-5 and 5-15 cm, which did not differ. Mineralized nitrogen at 5 cm was 25 % higher than at 15 cm (P<0.001).The equation used to describe the increase in mineralization over time was adequate, since it showed a good fit (R2>0.9) (Table 3). In all cases the exponential growth was stable, as shown in Figures 1, 2 and 3. The presence of the legume increased N mineralization in S5 and S8, but not in S3 as in the ANA incubation. Soils with Arachis. pintoi with 5 and 8 years produced more mineralized N (207 and 208 µg) than in native pasture soils (166 and 109 µg). Anaerobic incubation showed that nitrogen (N) mineralization was higher in the arable layer (0-5 cm) than at 5-15 cm. Soil depth was definitely the most important factor in explaining the differences in nitrogen (N) mineralization: soils 0-5 cm mineralized 104±7.0 μg versus soils 5-15 cm deep (70±5.4 μg). This difference is equivalent to one-third more N mineralized in the arable layer, which can be explained by the contribution of leaf litter to the soil surface. In the case of sites with Arachis. pintoi, a large volume of roots can be found at 5-10 cm depth (personal observation). These results coincide with data from temperate zones, where the maximum mineralization accumulated in the upper layer (0-18 cm) represented 42 % of the total mineralized N, compared to that found at 18-108 cm depth (22). No clear trend in nitrogen (N) mineralization was observed with age of Arachis. pintoi in pastures. At the 0-5 cm depth in 3-year-old Arachis. pintoi, the soil mineralized 131 μg,compared to the 5 (248 μg) and 8 (239 μg) year-old sites. This omission in trends was also observed in the ANA results (Table 2). On average at 0-5 cm, the soil with A. pintoi mineralized 46 % less nitrogen (N) than soils with older pastures, which could be due to the fact that sites with 5- and 8-year-old Arachis. pintoi maintained a higher legume cover (85 and 100 %), which allowed a greater amount of plant material to be degraded.Also, Arachis pintoi developed a greater root volume (22.6±22.6 g; 2 kg capacity pot), which may have contributed, over time, to a greater release of nitrogen (N) to the system.In Carimagua, Colombia, during the dry season and in clay soil, it has been observed that after 100 days, the roots of Arachis pintoi lose more carbon (65%) and nitrogen (70%) than Brachiaria humidicola (38 and 26%) and B. decumbens (32 and 12%)(19).If nitrogen (N) mineralization is correlated with soil N content, then nitrogen (N)-poor sites release fewer inorganic ions than nitrogen (N)-rich areas in a given time interval (25); although better substrates tend to have higher productivity, which translates into more efficient nitrogen (N) cycling (26). In coastal soils of Washington and Oregon states, a positive correlation (R2=0.89) was found between soil N content (0.09 to 0.40%) and N mineralization rate (0.9 to 45.5 μg N g-1 soil d-1) (27). In our study, the soils used were low in N (Table 1), and mineralization values had a low correlation with soil N content: R2=0.30 and 0.29 for sites with A. pintoi at 0-5 and 5-15 cm. These differences in R2 could probably be associated with other soil factors, such as the chemical nature of the organic matter, the species and age of the plant material, the particle size of the plant residues, the nitrogen (N) content of the residue, the carbon:N ratio of the residue, and the type and amount of clay present. In general, soluble organic materials with simple molecular structures, young legumes, residues with high N content, and a low carbon: nitrogen (N) ratio decompose more rapidly (28). Table 3. Simple exponential equations fitted with approximation to the maximum value for mineralized N (Y) at a certain time (X) in soil samples taken from sites established at different ages with or without Arachis pintoi (Ap), and their correlation coefficients associated within a native pasture (3 años- Arachis. pintoi), and the last one, with African star - Cynodon nlemfuensis- (5 años- A. pintoi) at the same time.

Table 1. Chemical components of control soils and soils from pastures with Arachis pintoi of 3, 5, 8 and 11 years old used to determine N mineralization.

Depth (cm)	Ph	%Nitrogen	Carbon %	Proportion CN	Nitrogen(N) %	Carbo no % no % no % no % no % no % no % no % no	C:N ratio
Cotrol 3 years Arachis pintoi 3 years							
0-5 5.50	5.5	0.13±0.00†	1.1±0.0	8.5	0.11±0.01	1.1±0.	10.0
5.15	5.65	0.10±0.00	1.1±0.00	8.5	0.11±0.01	1.1±0.	10.0
15-30	5.70	0.08±0.00	1.1±0.00	13.8	0.06±0.00	1.1±0.	18.3
Control year 5 Arachis. pintoi year 5							
0-5	5.50	0.18±0.01	1.9±0.04	10.6	0.18±0.02	1.9±0.	10.0
5-15	5.65	0.12±0.01	1.3±0.07	10.8	0.11±0.00	1.3±0.07	11.8
15-30	5.70	0.09±0.01	1.0±0.09	11.1	0.08±0.00	1.0±0.05	12.5
Control year 8 Arachis . pintoi year 8							
0-5	5.55	0.25±0.01	2.8±0.16	11.2	0.24±0.03	2.6±0.	10.8
0-5	5.55	0.25±0.01	2.8±0.16	11.1	0.08±0.00	2.6±0.	10.8
5-15	5.70	0.16±0.01	1.6±0.13	10.0	0.16±0.01	1.6±0.	10.0
Control year 11 Arachis. pintoi year11							
0-5	5.45	0.12±0.01	1.1±0.00	9.2 10.0	0.13±0.00	1.3±0.	10.0
5-15	5.66	0.08±0.01	1.1±0.00	13.8 10.0	0.09±0.01	0.9±0.	10.0
15-30	5.74	0.04±0.00	1.0±0.00	25.0 10.0	0.05±0.03	0.5±0.04	10.0

At sites S8 and S11, A. pintoi was sown in monoculture as seed banks. The legume was not inoculated, but in the four sites, a profuse inoculation of rhizobia of native strains was observed. The control areas corresponded to soils with native vegetation dominated by grasses of the genera Paspalum, Axonopus and Cynodon; and by legumes (<10 % of the area) mainly of the genera Desmodium and Calopogonium, which were under rotational grazing at the time of sampling, except for the control S8, which remained unused.The S11 control remained grazed until two years prior to sampling. Soils were unfertilized Ultisols for at least five years prior to and during the experiment.The site for each treatment was divided into four plots and a soil subsample was obtained from each plot using a auger. The four sub-samples for each depth were mixed to form a composite sample. Sampling depths were 0-5, 5-15 and 15-30 cm for anaerobic incubation (ANA), and 0-5 and 5-15 cm for aerobic incubation (AER). To determine the nitrogen (N) released by the anaerobic incubation method (ANA), a modification of the technique of Waring and Bremner (14) was used. Ten g of dry soil were weighed, placed in test tubes, to which 15 ml of distilled water was added. The tubes were sealed and kept at 40 °C for seven days (time 7). At the end of the incubation, ammonium was extracted by adding 30 ml of 3M KCl to the soils. The samples were shaken and filtered prior to NH4 + analysis by colorimetry with an autoanalyzer. The same procedure was performed prior to incubation to determine mineral N a time zero. To calculate the N released, the following formula was used (15):

Potential N mineralization rate=

(µg NH4 +-N g-1 soil, time 7 days) - (µg NH4 +-N g-1 soil, time 0 days)/7 days. To develop the aerobic incubation method (AER), soil samples (60 g) of 0-5 and 5-15 cm depth, from sites S3, S5 and S8, and their corresponding control treatments, were placed in columns (tubes of 3 cm diameter, 25 cm long) at 28 °C. At baseline, and subsequently at 7, 21, 49, 114, 231 and 301 days of incubation, the soils were percolated with 150 ml (in 50 ml increments) of a solution containing 1 mM MgSO4, 1 mM CaCl2,0.9 mM KCl and 0.1 mM KH2PO4 (16). Ammonium and nitrate were analyzed by colorimetry with an autoanalyzer, according to the following equation (15): mineralized N= (µg NO3+NH4 sample - µg NO3+NH4 blank)/g soil. Data from both experiments were analyzed separately, as a split-plot design using soils (with or without the legume) as the major plot and depths as subplots, repeated four (ANA) or three (AER) times.Analyses of variance were performed using mineralization rates and accumulated mineralized N as response variables. Comparisons of means were made using DMS. To describe mineralization trends, the data were fitted(17) to simple exponential curves approximating the maximum value. To choose the equation that best described the trends, the R2 value was used as a criterion, and the equation chosen was: Y = y0 + a(1-e-bx) Where Y is the mineralized Nitrogen at time x; y0 is the mineralized Nitrogen when x = 0; a is the asymptote or maximum mineralized Nitrogen, reached as x → ∞; and b is the rate of Nitrogen mineralization. Anaerobic incubation

RESULTS

The ANA results were atypical and inconsistent. The highest mineralization rate was expected in soils planted with the introduced legume, rather than with the native pasture, where on these sites the native legume population has been estimated to be very poor (7.1 %)(18). Mineralization data will always correspond to µg NH4 +-N g-1 soil d-1.Considering the ANA results, in S3 there were differences in anaerobic potential mineralization between pastures with A. pintoi and its control, at the three depths (Table 2). The average of the three depths was 3.1±0.7 (pastures with A. pintoi) vs. 10.4±1.3 µg (native pastures) (P<0.001); the latter value was three times higher than the mineralized soil N in the pasture with A. pintoi.Mineralization was higher at 0-5 cm depth, and different (P<0.001) at the other depths. The interaction soil (with or without legume) by depth was not significant (P>0.05).In S5 the differences in anaerobic mineralization between native pasture soils (6.2±1.4 µg) and soils with the legume (7.5±1.5 µg) were not significant (Table 2). In all cases the mineralization rate decreased with depth, averaging for both soils (with and without the forage legume) 10.6±1.8, 6.1±1.5 and 3.1± 0.7 µg (P≤0.05) at 0-5, 5-15 and 15-30 cm. Only in S5 at 0-5cm there was a slightly higher value compared to native pasture soil (11.6 vs. 10.6 µg), respectively. As in S5, N mineralized from site S8 with A. pintoi was not significantly different from native pasture soil (8.9±2.3 µg) and with A. pintoi (6.5±1.9 µg); however, there were significant differences (P≤0.001) between 0-5 cm (14.4±3.1) and the shallowest depths (5.7±0.6 and 3.1±1.0 µg at 5-15 and 15-30 cm). At S11, the control showed a high N mineralization rate (9.0±1.4 µg), different (P<0.001) from the soil with A. pintoi (3.3±0.8 µg). The effect of soil depth as well as the interaction with pasture was, in both cases, highly significant (P<0.001).In the nutrient uptake process, the rhizosphere is very important, particularly under low fertility conditions; and fibrous grass roots affect N mineralization (19). In S11 these results were even more unexpected, since the site had a legume cover close to 100 %; however, the control produced 2.7 times more mineral N than the soil with the introduced legume. In S5 and S8 the pastures with A. pintoi produced on average 6.3±1.1 µg , which is only 70 % of the N produced by the soil with native pasture alone (9.0±5.7 µg). In the Cerrado brasileño, data on potential N mineralization (incubation at 40 °C, 7 d) in various land-use systems, ranging from native pastures (savanna) to continuous cropping systems on Oxisols soils(20) have shown that, contrary to our results, potentially mineralizable N was highest in associated Brachiaria decumbens/Stylosanthes guianensis pastures (63 kg N ha-1), followed by Brachiaria decumbens alone (43 kg N ha-1), no-till continuous cropping (26 kg N ha-1), native savanna (23 kg N ha-1) and continuous cropping with conventional tillage (18 kg N ha-1). These authors mentioned that the presence of the legume promoted microbial activity, and therefore more N was mineralized. Other authors found that the introduction of Stylosanthes spp. in an Andropogon gayanus pasture had a positive effect on potentially mineralizable N. They estimated that the associated pasture had a positive effect on N mineralization. They estimated that the associated pasture, at a soil depth of 0-5 cm, produced 20.3 µg N g-1 soil, compared to the grass pasture alone (11.6 µg N g-1 soil)(21). In our study, the trend of decreasing N mineralization with depth was consistent across all sites, although correlation coefficients (R2) between soil depth and mineralization were not high: 0.36 and 0.50 for sites with A. pintoi and native pasture, respectively. Several studies have shown that net N mineralization decreases with increasing depth, and have mentioned that above 20 cm it accounts for as much as 75 %(22) or 61 %(23) of the total. However, the relative importance of net mineralization from the subsoil can be high during dry periods, when moisture limitations are present in the surface layer, but not in the subsoil (24).

Anaerobic mineralization rates (µg NH4-N g-1 soil d-1) of soil samples from 3-, 5-, 8- and 11-year-old pastures with A. pintoi and their corresponding sites (control).

Years with Arachis pintoi or control	Soil depth cm 0-5 5-15 15-30		
3 Arachi pintoi	5.8 ± 1.3	2.4 ± 0.2	1.0 ± 0.1
Control	15.1 ± 2.9	10.2 ± 1.2	6.0 ± 0.5
5 Arachis pintoi	11.6 ± 2.6	3.3 ± 2.33	3.5 ± 1.0
Control	10.7 ± 2.4	7.7 ± 2.5	2.7 ± 0.7
8 Arachis pintoi	14.5 ± 3.3	6.0 ± 1.2	1.9 ± 0.7
Control	18.7 ± 4.4	6.0 ± 0.6	4.2 ± 1.8
11 Arachis pintoi	6.7 ± 1.3	2.3 ± 0.4	0.9 ± 0.1
Control	15.1 ± 2.7	7.8 ± 1.1	4.2 ± 0.9

Aerobic N mineralization accumulated in soil samples at two depths in 3-year-old Arachis pintoi pastures and its control site.

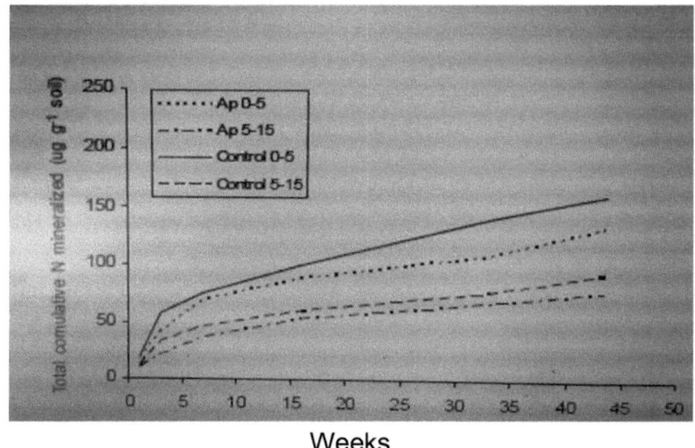

Aerobic N mineralization accumulated in soil samples at two depths in 5-year-old A. pintoi pastures and its control site.

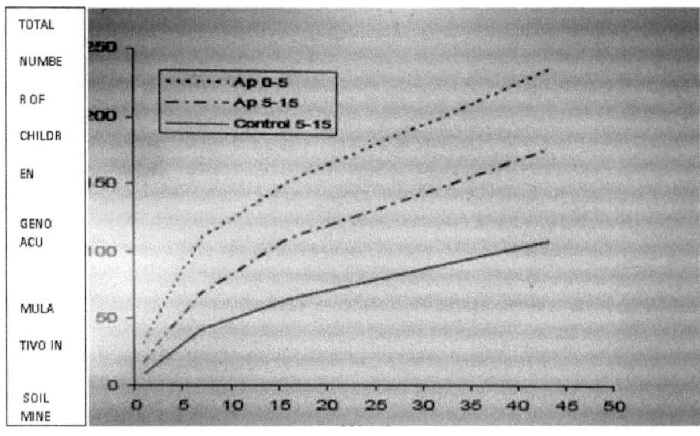

Weeks

Aerobic N mineralization accumulated in soil samples at two depths in 8-year-old A. pintoi pastures and its control site.

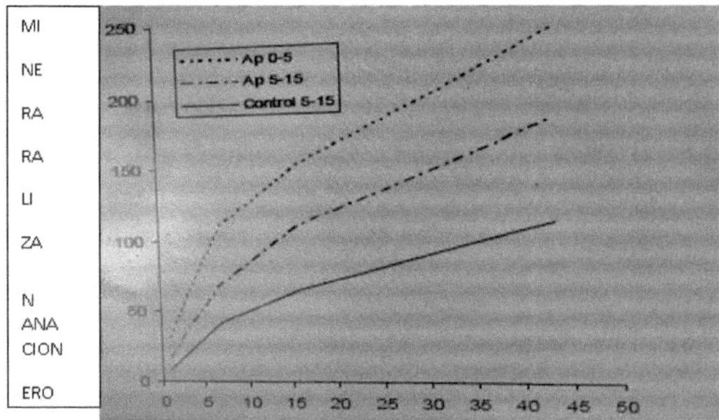

Weeks

Table 3. Simple exponential equations fitted with approximation to the maximum value for mineralized N (Y) at a certain time (X) in soil samples taken from established sites at different ages with or without pintoi (Ap), and their correlation coefficients.

Site Arachis pintoi by year	Soil depth (cm)	Arachis pintoi sites.	R2	Control sites	R2
	0-5	Y=15.2+111.5 (1-e-0.076x)	0.94	Y=24.8+145.6(1-e–0.052x)	0.94
5	0-15	Y=6.72+71.2(1-e-0.068x)	0.98	Y=11.9+78.6 (1-e-0.067x)	0.93
5	0.5	Y=30.2+264.3 (1-e-0.035x)	0.94	Y=27.4+225.5 (1-e-0.032x)	0.96
5	5-15	Y=13.0+158.8 (1-e-0.054x)	0.96	Y=17.1+129.2 (1-e-0.041x)	0.97
	0.5	Y=25.2+225.3 (1-e-0.056x)	0.98	n.a	
	5-15	Y=11.4+185.0 (1-e-0.048x)	0.99	Y=5.7+118.9 (1-e-0.044x)	0.98

n.a.= Equation not available.

LITERATURE CITED

1. Améndola R, Castillo E, Martínez PA. Forage resource profiles. In: FAO editor. Country Pasture Profiles. Rome, Italy. 2005 [on line]. http://www.fao.org/agp/agpc/doc/counprof/Mexico/Mexico.htm. Accessed May 8, 2007.

2. Westerhof R, Vilela L, Ayarza MA, Zech W. Labile N and the nitrogen management index of Oxisols in the Brazilian Cerrados. In: Thomas R, Ayarza MA editors. Sustainable land managementfor the Oxisols of the Latin American savannas. Cali, Colombia: International Center for Tropical Agriculture, CIAT publicationNo. 312, 1999:133-140.

3. Rao I, Ayarza MA, Thomas RJ, Fisher MJ, Sanz JI, Spain JM,Lascano CE. Soil plant factors and processes affecting productivityin ley farming. In: Hardy B editor. Pastures for the tropical lowlands. CIATs contribution. Cali, Colombia: CIAT publication No. 211, 1992:145-175.

4. Humphreys LR. Environmental adaptation of tropical pasture plants. 1st ed. London, UK: Macmillan Publishers Ltd; 1981.

5. Silvestre-Bradley R. Rhizobium inoculation trials designed to support a tropical forage legume selection programme. Plant and Soil 1984;(82):377-386.

6. Giller K. Cadisch G. Future benefits from biological nitrogen fixation: An ecological approach on agriculture. Plant and Soil 1995;(174):225-277.

7. Thomas RJ, Asakawa NM, Rondon MA, Alarcon HF. Nitrogen fixation by tree tropical forage legumes in an acid-soil savanna of Colombia. Soil Biol Biochem 1997;(29):801-808.

8. Valles B. Contribution of the forage legume Arachis pintoi to soil fertility in a tropical pasture system in Veracruz, Mexico. [doctoral thesis]. Wye, Ashford, Kent, UK: Imperial College of Science Technology and Medicine, University of London; 2001.

9. Thomas RJ, Asakawa NM. Decomposition of leaf-litter from tropical forage grasses and legumes. Soil Biol Biochem 1993;(25):1351-1361.

10. Abreu OC, Scotti-Muzzi MR, Abrantes-Purcino H, Evodio- Marriel I, Horta-de Sa N.M. Decomposition of Arachis pintoi and Hyparrhenia rufa litters in monoculture and intercropped systems under lowland soil. Pesq Agrop Bras 2003;(38):1089 1095.

11. Toledo JM. Tropical legume research plan for CIEEGT. Consultancy Report, FAO Project: MEX 1781015 (restricted circulation document). Martinez de la Torre, Veracruz, Mexico. 1986.

12. Hernández T, Valles B, Castillo E. Evaluation of grasses and forage legumes in Veracruz, Mexico. Valles B, Castillo E, Hernández T. Seasonal production of forage legumes in Veracruz, Mexico. Past Trop 1992;(14):32-36.

14. Waring SA, Bremner JM. Ammonium production in soil under waterlogged conditions as an index of nitrogen availability. Nature 1964;(201):951-952.

15. Anderson JM, Ingram JSI. Tropical soil biology and fertility: A handbook of methods. 2nd ed. Wallingford, UK: CAB International; 1993. 16. Cassman KG, Munns DN. Nitrogen mineralization as affected by soil-moisture, temperature, and depth. Soil Sci Soc Am J 1980;(44):1233-1237.

17. SPSS. Statistical Package for the Social Sciences. Sigma Plot for Windows Version 4.00. Chicago, Ill, USA: SPSS Inc; 1997.
18. Bosman HG, Castillo E, Valles B, De Lucía GR. Botanical composition and nodulation of legumes in native pastures of the coastal plain of the Gulf of Mexico. Past Trop 1990; 12(1):1-8.
19. Gijsman AJ, Alarcón HF, Thomas RJ. Root decomposition on tropical grasses and legumes, as affected by soil texture and season. Soil Biol Biochem 1997;(29):1443-1450.

20. Fuhrmann S, Neufeldt H, Westerhof R, Ayarza M, da Silva JE, Zech W. Soil organic carbon, carbohydrates, amino sugars, and potentially mineralizable nitrogen under different land-use systems in Oxisols of the Brazilian Cerrados. In: Thomas R, Ayarza MA editors. Sustainable land management for the Oxisols of the Latin American savannas. Cali, Colombia: International Center for Tropical Agriculture, CIAT publication No. 312; 1999:110-122.
21. Cadisch G, Carvalho EF, Suhet AR, Vilela L, Soares W, Spain JM, Urquiaga S, Giller KE, Boddey RM. Importance of legume nitrogen fixation in sustainability of pastures in the Cerrados of Brazil. In: Baker MJ editor. Proc XVII International Grassland Congress 1993, Palmerston North, New Zealand.1993:1915-1916.
22. Kandeler E, Eder G, Sobotik M. Microbial biomass, N mineralization, and the activities of various enzymes in relation to nitrate leaching and root distribution in a slurry-amended grassland. Biol Fert Soils 1994; 18(1):7-12. 23. Hadas A, Feigenbaum S, Feigin A, Portnoy R. Nitrogen mineralization in profiles of differently managed soil types. Soil Sci Soc Am J 1986;(50):314-319.

24. Rovira P, Vallejo VR. Organic carbon and nitrogen mineralization under mediterranean climatic conditions: the effects of incubation depth. Soil Biol Biochem 1997;(29):1509-1520.
25. Alexander M. Introduction to soil microbiology. 2nd ed. New York, USA: John Wiley and Sons; 1977. 26. Reich PB, Grigal DF, Aber JD, Gower ST. Nitrogen mineralization and productivity in 50 hardwood and conifer stands on diverse soils. Ecology 1997;(78):335-347.
27. Prescott CE, Chappell HN, Vesterdal L. Nitrogen turnover in forest floors of Coastal Douglas-Fir at sites differing in soil nitrogen capital. Ecology 2000;(81):1878-1886. 28. Whitehead DC. Grassland Nitrogen. 1st ed. Wallingford, Oxon, UK; CAB International; 1995.
29. Gilliam FS, Lyttle NL, Thomas A, Adams MB. Soil variability along a nitrogen mineralization and nitrification gradient in a nitrogen-saturated Hardwood forest. Soil Sci Soc Am J 2005;(69):247-256.

30. Neill C, Piccolo MC, Melillo JM, Steudler PA, Cerri CC. Nitrogen dynamics in Amazon forest and pasture soils measured by 15N pool dilution. Soil Biol Biochem 1999;(31):567-572.

31. Trinsoutrot I, Recous S, Bentz B, Lineres M, Cheneby D, NicolardoB. T Biochemical quality of crop residues and carbon and nitrogen mineralization kinetics under nonlimiting nitrogen conditions. Soil Sci Soc Am J 2000;(64):918-926.

32. Collins A, Allinson DW. Nitrogen mineralization in soil from perennial grassland measured through long-term laboratory incubations. J Agric Sci 2002;(138):301-310.

33. Munevar F, Wollum AG. Effects of the addition of phosphorus and inorganic nitrogen on carbon and nitrogen mineralization in Andepts from Colombia. Soil Sci Soc Am J 1977;(41):540-545.

34. Cadisch G, Giller KE, Urquiaga S, Miranda CHB, Boddey RM, Schunke RM. Does phosphorus supply enhance soil N mineralization in Brazilian pastures? Eur J Agron 1994;(3):339-345.

35. Whitehead DC. Nutrient elements in grassland: Soil-plant-animal relationships. 1st ed. Wallingford, UK: CAB International; 2000.

36. Cadisch G, Giller KE. Soil organic matter management: The role of residues quality in C sequestration and N supply. In: Rees RM, Ball BC, Campbell CD, Watson CA editors. Sustainable management of soil organic matter. 1st ed. Wallingford, Oxon, UK; CAB International; 2001. 990;(12):29.

More Books!

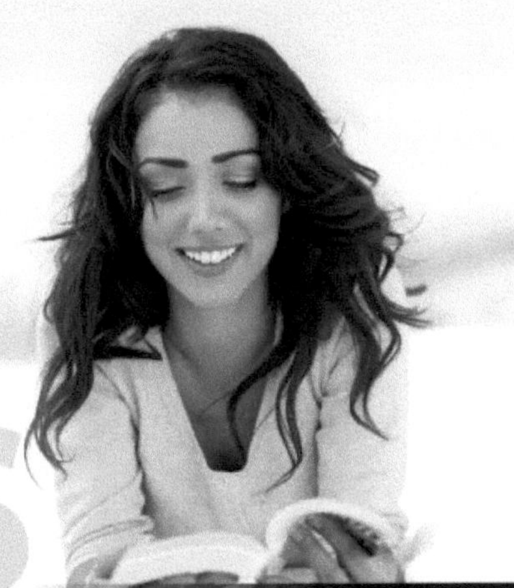

yes

I want morebooks!

Buy your books fast and straightforward online - at one of world's fastest growing online book stores! Environmentally sound due to Print-on-Demand technologies.

Buy your books online at
www.morebooks.shop

Kaufen Sie Ihre Bücher schnell und unkompliziert online – auf einer der am schnellsten wachsenden Buchhandelsplattformen weltweit! Dank Print-On-Demand umwelt- und ressourcenschonend produzi ert.

Bücher schneller online kaufen
www.morebooks.shop

info@omniscriptum.com
www.omniscriptum.com

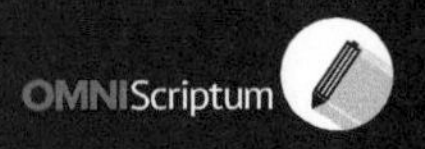

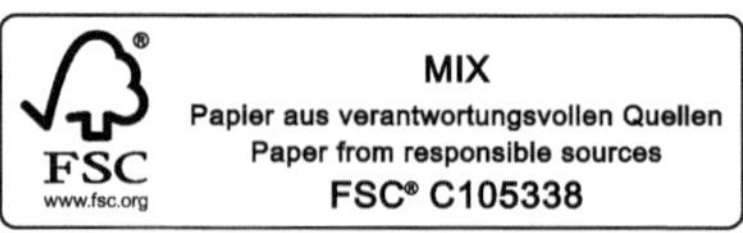

MIX
Papier aus verantwortungsvollen Quellen
Paper from responsible sources
FSC® C105338
FSC
www.fsc.org

Printed by Books on Demand GmbH, Norderstedt / Germany